Finding The Bloom Of The

Cactus
Generation

Improving the quality of life for Seniors

Maggie Walters
2007

Maggie Walters

Published 2007
LIFESUCCESS PUBLISHING, LLC
8900 E Pinnacle Peak Road, Suite D240
Scottsdale, AZ 85255

Telephone:	800.473.7134
Fax:	480.661.1014

E-mail:	admin@lifesuccesspublishing.com
ISBN:	1-59930-011-5
Cover:	Chris Mackey & LifeSuccess Publishing
Layout:	Lloyd Arbour & LifeSuccess Publishing

COMPANIES, ORGANIZATIONS, INSTITUTIONS, AND INDUSTRY PUBLICATIONS: Quantity discounts are available on bulk purchases of this book for reselling, educational purposes, subscription incentives, gifts, sponsorship, or fundraising. Special books or book excerpts can also be created to fit specific needs such as private labeling with your logo on the cover and a message from a VIP printed inside. For more information please contact our Special Sales Department at LifeSuccess Publishing.

Medical Disclaimer

The information contained in this book is provided for your general information only. Neither LifeSuccess Publishing, LLC nor the author, Maggie Walters provide medical advice or engage in the practice of medicine. LifeSuccess Publishing, LLC and Maggie Walters do not recommend particular medical treatments for any individual. For questions regarding your medical condition LifeSuccess Publishing, LLC and Maggie Walters recommend that you consult your physician or health care professional before pursuing any course of treatment.

For Diana and Caroline

Acknowledgements

I would like to thank the patient souls who put up with my nagging questions and without whom this book would be less: Alexandra De Avalon, Dr. Mary Clark, Harriet Goslins, and Lansing Barrett Gresham. A special thank you goes to Dr. Cecil Cutting for contributing the forward to this book. Thank you also to all of my clients, their families and the staff at the care facilities for being who they are.

I also want to thank the team at LifeSuccess Publishing whose support and encouragement moved this project forward.

Especially thank you to my inspiring daughters whose creativity and strength have helped me to find my voice.

Foreword
by Dr. Cecil Cutting

In *Cactus Generation,* the author shares with us her years of experience and interest in improving the lives of the aging population. Perhaps she can pierce the capsule of isolation that enshrouds the aging dementia or Alzheimer victim. Perhaps she can reach a few viable neurons ready for recognition or ready to escape the wild tangles or forgotten memories. Perhaps she can provide a moment of trust and calm.

We are all aware of the increasing number of seniors in our population. Caring for the aging will be an increasing challenge both for the nation and for the individual; both economically and socially. We anxiously await scientific achievement to provide relief.

In the meantime, those of is who have loved ones who have fallen victim to dementia are acutely aware of its complexity and the multitude of questions it generates. Will she be best cared for at home or in a custodial facility; guilt in sending her; medication; what does she remember; do visits help or agitate; does she feel alone; abandoned or is she resigned; what is left in her mind and can it be reached; what can be done to help?

As efficient and professional as the nursing staff may be, they have little time to sit down with a patient to build a trust that might open up the gates of insight into another world.

Maggie Walters is dedicated to bridge that gap. She describes energies (chi) that help. Certainly there are energies that reinforce communication: the warmth of the body, the touch, the smell, the sound of a reassuring voice, the understanding and trust that can be built.

Maggie has been seeing my wife at a custodial facility for several years. I am convinced that her communication skills and the trust she has built has been a comfort and a reassurance to my wife and I am sure it has been for me as well.

Dr. Cutting graduated from Stanford Medical School in 1935. He has had a long career as a surgeon and a medical group administrator. He was a co-founder of the Kaiser Permanente medical care program.

Contents

Introduction

During the past few years there seems to have been
an increase in the amount of talk about aging and seniors.
Disturbing reports in the press hint that we, as a society, will
not be able to afford to take care of our aging population.
In previous generations, there was never much talk about
seniors. They might qualify for a discount on the bus or at
the ball game. Occasionally someone's grandmother would
show up, closely shepherded by a son or daughter. Otherwise,
they seemed to just disappear. On the odd occasion when a
senior or someone in a wheelchair appeared, no one knew
how to relate to them. More recently, nearly everyone I meet
seems to have a story about an elderly relative. I casually
mentioned to Russ, my service agent at the auto dealership,
I was writing this book and he immediately began telling me
about his grandmother. He knew that her health was an issue
for his family and I find most people are focused on one thing
or another relating to care for their older person. "Is this
becoming a burden?" I ask. Sometimes they admit they are
feeling that way, sometimes not. They almost always say there
is a problem and their story goes on.

Those born during the population explosion at the end of
the Second World War, referred to as the baby boomers (born
between 1940 and 1960), are fast approaching the age when they
will fall into the senior category. There are many of them and
they are living longer than previous generations. When they can
no longer care for themselves, will their families or society be
able to care for them? The American Geriatrics Society reports

that baby boomers, as they age and reach retirement, "…are expected to have a major impact on the health and social service systems of the United States."[1] "What will we do with them?" seems to be the question on everyone's lips. This question has given birth to the concept of 'long-term care.'

Long-term care is now the hot topic. More and more agents are specializing in this type of insurance with their market expanding as the boomers age. The focus of the pitch is on the cost of long-term care that nearly everyone will inevitably need. Whereas in 2000, there were 35 million people over the age of sixty-five, by 2030 that population is expected to reach 70 million. These figures compute to one in every five people.[2] In 1995, approximately 12.8 million people in the United States needed some form of long-term care. Although this figure includes institutional care as well as community-based and home care, frequently offered by unpaid friends or relatives, at that time the majority of people, over 10 million, were receiving care either at home or in a community setting.[3] Ten years later, formal long-term care facilities have sprung up nationwide.

The group aged eighty-five and older, termed 'the oldest old,' is the fastest growing segment of our population and is the most in need of long-term care, due primarily to chronic conditions.[4] These conditions range from physical limitations restricting their capacity to perform normal 'activities of daily living' (ADL) to cognitive failures, both of which lead to the need for constant supervision. The need for formal institutional care rises with age. At age 85 there is a 49% chance of spending time in a care facility. By 2020, an estimated 14 million of the elderly will require some form of long-term care and 3.6 million people will be in need of formal nursing care.[5] There are 75,883 long-term care facilities in the United States, including senior housing residences, and of those 15,989 are licensed skilled nursing facilities.[6] Many have special units to care for Alzheimer's and other dementia patients. Does this sound like enough?

There does seem to be general agreement that the current situation surrounding long- term care has numerous problems such as finance, choice and availability of care situations and pressure felt by families and caregivers.[7] I do not intend to address financial or any other issue relating to the development or organization of the long-term care system. My sole purpose is to discuss the quality of life for those vanishing seniors and how families, caregivers and society can continue to relate to them as they move toward the inevitable end of life.

This is a true story is about working with seniors in a care facilities. Identities have been changed to protect privacy. The situation presented itself through necessity, not by design, and the journey makes an important contribution toward understanding the observations and rewards of the work. I hope readers who relate to this story will feel a sense of relief in finding that they are not in this alone and will find ways to help and support their senior through this most difficult time of life. This book is about finding means of support, other than financial, for the senior population through connection on many levels. Support is about relationship and witnessing a life nearing completion. In the process of giving support we clarify our own inner values as well as those of our elders. A connection can be established which affects both you and your senior. It increases our understanding and appreciation of life – every minute of it – and opens a doorway through which we can join the network of all living things. Seniors have rich experiences which can enhance our value and meaning of life, if only we would let them.

Chapter 1

Growing Up Older

People grow up in various circumstances and surroundings and by the end of the physical "growing up" period, you are considered an adult. Being an adult in the physical sense is quite different from being an adult mentally or emotionally. Some people remain children, emotionally, until well into their adult years. Some never grow up at all. The ideal situation is for all parts of you to mature at the same time. That rarely seems to happen. Maybe the real grown-ups are older souls who have lived previous lives and their spirits know what to expect. They seem to emotionally adjust more easily and relate to the world and their responsibilities in an adult manner. Of course, to accept that, you have to believe in multiple lives. It may be a stretch to believe in more than one life, however it would certainly explain a lot of conundrums. Sometimes we think we are grown up and sometimes, although we have grown up, we are not older at all; we are still children.

Stretching north along Lake Michigan, the older suburbs of Chicago were inhabited by graceful homes with sweeping porches and brick walkways. The sidewalks were uneven where the roots of the giant trees had pushed up the corners of the paving blocks. The Northwestern Railroad line ran along the shore giving commuters quick access to the city. The train ran on the wrong side of the track so if you didn't know you could easily be waiting on the opposite platform only to watch the engine pull in on the other side. The sign at Kenilworth Station was scripted with a sweeping initial K underlining the other letters. As with many suburban towns there was a right side and a wrong side of the tracks. The larger homes shrank in stature and were closer together as they moved further west, ultimately turning into ranch style houses in cul-de-sacs.

Virginia Kress Goodrich grew up in a square white house with a single stall garage attached on one side. Her parents, Martin and Alice Kress, hoped to move to one of the more imposing houses east of the tracks but Virginia didn't notice their aspirations until she was much older. The original house was on a very straight street lined with similar houses and large elm trees. The trees were beautiful although Dutch elm disease was often whispered and without the trees the street would certainly have been less appealing. All the streets bore the names of trees and the Kress's street was the last one in a long line descending from a ridge and ending at the street at the bottom of the hill beyond which there were more streets with more houses. The family house was near the bottom but Virginia wasn't allowed to go past the corner. There was some mystery about what was around there. She could see the back of the house on the corner and a boy about her age lived there but he didn't go to her school. She overheard her mother say he was a problem child because his parents were often away and he was left with the housekeeper, so he had to go to a special school. Even though he lived so close, she didn't know him very well. Her best friend lived in the house directly behind her and, whenever they played with the boy on the corner, he always did something they considered disgusting. Any attention was better than none.

Virginia was an only child and even though she had neighborhood and school friends, she spent a lot of time by herself. She watched *Mickey Mouse Club* and wanted to be Annette, so pretty and popular. One year she secretly sent away for ears. Virginia made up games and imaginary friends with whom she had lengthy conversations. Mostly, she wanted to be a cowboy. It was the days of the *Lone Ranger* and the *Cisco Kid*. One year, she received chaps and a cowboy hat for

Christmas and spent many hours galloping around the back yard, making trails in the leaves and jumping across make-believe ravines. Her parents didn't interrupt her solitary games and she was happy enough. She always respected her parents and accepted their wishes never daring to disagree or have an opinion of her own. She sought approval from her mother more than anyone because she seemed to have the power in the family. Her father was more easy-going, sociable and liked by everyone. This relationship with her parents fostered a difficult situation in later years.

The Kresses were a small family. Martin and Alice each had one sibling but the family didn't see either of them very often. Growing up, Virginia never saw her cousins, her uncle's children. She was in high school before she even knew she had real cousins - other than a mystery one who always seemed to be in trouble. They were not her age, did not live close and there seemed to be no reason to get together with them. Virginia would hear about her friends' families from time to time. Sometimes, they would be visiting grandparents and she always thought that sounded like fun, although she had no conception of what it would be like. Her grandparents, with the exception of her paternal grandmother, had died before she was born. Alice used to tell stories about her father, Virginia's grandfather, and he sounded like a fun person. He had lived in a small town somewhere in the north and had held a number of city and county offices. In old photos, he and his friends were dressed up in funny outfits. They would go out into the surrounding countryside and dig up artifacts that had been buried long ago in tribal ceremonies. Although this behavior would be considered a sacrilege today, it was common in those times. Virginia's grandfather enjoyed travel and always went to Florida in the winter to get away from the cold weather and storms. She never knew him and her grandmother, who had died many years before, was never mentioned.

Virginia's paternal grandmother, Grandmother Kress, as she was called, lived about twenty miles away, but the family rarely saw her. Her husband, Virginia's other grandfather, had died years before. He had been the dean of a small college and there were many stories about the trouble Martin and his brother got into trying to embarrass their father in front of the students. Virginia recalled the story about how, in their teenage years, the two boys had shared a car. Each painted his side of the vehicle a different color. One time they were chased by the police who failed to spot the car because they passed it on the wrong side. Martin had a strap taken to him on more than one occasion when he behaved particularly badly. Nevertheless, it sounded like Grandfather Kress had a sense of humor and Virginia thought she would have liked him. Alice always said Martin and his mother were too much alike and that was why they didn't get along well. Martin's brother, Uncle Eddy, also lived nearby, but the family hardly ever saw him either. As a child Virginia imagined the two of them getting together and talking about her. Not only did she not have much contact with her one grandmother, her family lived in community of other young families who also did not seem to have grandparents or, if they did, no one ever saw them.

The few times Grandmother Kress did come to visit, never at holidays such as Thanksgiving or Christmas, Virginia remembered as being rather scary. She was definitely not huggable and sitting on her lap was out of the question. In fact, it never even occurred to Virginia who was to keep a respectful distance and be very quiet. Grandmother Kress was a tall lady with glasses and curled white hair that never moved. She stood very erect and looked kind of bony with a stern set jaw and thin lips that barely parted when she spoke. Her hands had big blue veins that looked like they might burst at any moment. She wore stiff looking clothing that buttoned tightly around her neck and she had a very scary way of looking down at Virginia through her spectacles. On one visit, she had a broken leg encased in a large white cast with her toes peeking out of the end and she used a stick to help her walk. This episode was more frightening than the others and stayed vividly in

Virginia's memory. She sat quietly on the back stoop guarding her wooden farm animals, horse and pig, and tried to make herself as small as possible. Grandmother Kress disappeared back to the city and was not thought of again for a long time. Martin rarely mentioned her.

As Martin and his brother did not get along very well, Aunt Rose, Alice's sister, was the only other adult in the family's life. She did not live near Chicago. Virginia primarily remembered her aunt as being alone because she had been widowed at a young age and she had no children. When Virginia was growing up, Aunt Rose visited the family twice a year as a stop-off place during her migration to Florida for the winter. Aunt Rose must have picked up this way of life from her father as she had cared for him when he was elderly and stayed close to him until he died. Alice was not very involved with her father's aging process because she had her own family to care for.

When Aunt Rose came to visit, she stayed in the guest room, right next to Virginia. In the morning, Virginia used to sneak in to see if she was awake yet because she was always curious to see what was in her aunt's suitcase. Aunt Rose loved to travel and see new places. She went around the world several times and visited exotic places with strange sounding names like Katmandu, a city Virginia would also visit as an adult. One time, Aunt Rose traveled down the Amazon River on a *raft*. On another occasion, she came back with many slides of native people with large stretched lips. The family watched the slides with attention and listened to the stories of her travels. Virginia was too young to relate to the exotic places and people, but she couldn't wait for Aunt Rose to arrive because she always brought presents. If she had just returned from a trip, the gifts could be rather unusual. The ornate silver elephant sat on a shelf because Virginia didn't know exactly how to play with it. The native jewelry was beautiful and too heavy and embarrassing to wear, but she always had candy and chocolates in her bag too. In her later years Aunt Rose took to traveling with the Arthur Murray Dance Studio because she loved to dance and it gave her companionship. Virginia didn't think of her aunt as an older person; she was always so full of enthusiasm and stories. She was a jolly, happy and active person who loved life to the end. She really never was *old*.

As a teen-ager, Virginia was shy and often came straight home after school to finish her homework so she would be allowed to watch television in the evening. Sometimes she would go to high school games but she liked swim meets best. The prom was a big event because she had a beautiful white dress with a sequined top and she was escorted by the boy from down the street. Holidays were the times when she wished she had a larger or extended family. Some years, the family would go to the home of friends of her parents for Christmas dinner. These friends had five children and with that many people around the table, the atmosphere seemed so jolly. Still, there were no grandparents in sight. Virginia was more concerned about what presents she would get than about how older or infirm people spent the holidays. This early atmosphere around elders did not foster an attitude of caring, respect or much of anything at all, other than perhaps fear. She certainly had no desire to touch an old person. Like a spiky cactus, they appeared to be prickly; her impression was that they were always bony, sometimes smelled bad, looked kind of vacant or talked nonsense. As she grew into her teens and twenties, she tended to avoid elderly people as much as possible.

Martin decided to retire from the rat race at a relatively young age. He had worked at an advertising agency downtown and had moved up nicely in the company so his stock options and severance check gave him a substantial lump sum. Alice was pleased because that meant they could spend more time together. Virginia was living far away when they suddenly announced that they had sold the family home and were moving to Florida. This move was not altogether surprising. Of all the states, Florida has the largest population over sixty-five as well as having the greatest number of retirees moving into the state,[8] and Alice's family had a history of spending winter months there. Nevertheless, Virginia was shocked, speechless and, although she had a home of her own, she felt a sense of abandonment, as though she had been thrown out. Of course, her parents had every right to make that decision by themselves, but Virginia felt she should have been consulted. They had never even discussed it with her! She realized later that was the way the family worked. They were a very small unit but they were all independent and, although Virginia's life choices had always been influenced to some degree by her parents' wishes, each family member made their own choices, good or bad. In some ways, that relationship put a distance between Virginia and her parents. Despite that, she always knew she was loved. Even though she lived far away, she never felt removed from her early relationships with her parents, still relying on their advice and seeking approval. She always remained connected.[9] That connection was to play itself out in a way she could not even imagine at this earlier stage in her life.

When Virginia's parents decided to make this move, her perception of them changed. They suddenly went from being part of the work force to being retirees. That put them in a different category and somehow aged them in her eyes. Now they were old people. *Should she treat them differently?* she wondered. She still expected to be waited on hand and foot when she went to visit them. Was she a guest or was she returning to childhood habits? She was never really sure. She was also not sure how different their lives were after that move. They were active in the community, going to concerts and the theatre and out with new friends. Martin had a part-time job and an office and was on the board of a foundation. Alice didn't seem to do much at all other than wait for her husband to take her somewhere. Alice had always been like that. She liked to read; she collected books; she loved the opera and spent time listening to recordings. They were always thrilled when Virginia came to visit with her family. The grandchildren were a delight for them, although as they grew older, the children's endless energy began to tire them out more and more. By the time they were ready to go home Martin and Alice were exhausted, but later, when Virginia would call, her parents would say the house was so quiet.

The Kress's lives continued without much change for years until they decided to move out of their Florida house into a retirement community. It was one of those staged places where they could go from their own three bedroom apartment with a full kitchen to assisted living quarters to full nursing, all within the same complex. *A good idea,* they said. *Planning ahead.* Virginia's view of them changed again. Now, when she visited, she noticed visible signs of them aging. They no longer picked her up at the airport. She had to rent a car or take a cab. They wanted to have dinner earlier and went to bed by 8:30 PM. They became a little more stooped and seemed a little shorter. Her mother, especially, had less energy and just looked older. Although she recognized the signs of aging, she never connected it with her parents' state of mind. They still seemed competent enough, but were they? Virginia learned later that fear of losing independence and increasing frailty is a big issue when it comes to aging. We start thinking about it long before it happens.[10]

The new retirement complex was on the other side of the state, many miles away from Martin and Alice's old community where they had friends and an interest in the activities of the city. John and Ruth, friends from their old building, had also moved into the same new community. Although they had been friends for years, they didn't see much of each other after the move. Both couples had become wrapped up in their own health problems and socializing was not a priority. They didn't make many new friends there, either. Virginia wondered if the move had been wise and if they would have been better off staying in the community where they knew more people. Her mother said the health care was better there and, by that stage, Martin was quite ill.

Her parents retained their self-sufficiency in the retirement community. They had a nice three-bedroom apartment with a kitchen and two baths. They didn't cook much because there was a dining room and a snack bar for lunch. They had two cars and drove to the nearby shopping center and to a multitude of doctors' appointments. The retirement community had a bus to drive residents around town but, as far as Virginia knew, they never used it. Her mother complained about having to wait around for all the old people to get on and off and having to stop and wait at different places. Not exactly the private limousine service she had in mind.

Although they had aged, Virginia's parents also seemed to be very aware of the other elderly people around them. When she was visiting, they used to tell her to watch out for other drivers. *They can't see; they pull out in front of you; they back out without looking; you always have to drive defensively.* Sometimes, they would point out a car with a very small person driving so the car appeared to be driving itself. People seem to get smaller with age. Alice herself was fairly short and soon fell into the category of the invisible driver. She joked about it anyway. She also laughed about a friend who lived in another retirement community where meals were regularly provided. She had arranged to have lunch with her friend only to arrive and be told that her friend had already eaten. The friend cheerfully had lunch again with Alice anyway. She had forgotten she had eaten the first time. Virginia never saw the humor in this predicament but her mother thought it was hilarious. Later in her life, Alice discovered how her friend felt.

One time when Virginia was visiting they were at the beach and her father announced he didn't want to sit next to a frail-looking elderly man, only to discover the man was a friend who had lost a lot of weight due to cancer. At the time Virginia couldn't tell if her father felt bad about the remark or not but later in his life her father found himself in a similar position. He also used to joke about not buying green bananas because he didn't know if he would be around long enough for them to ripen, and her mother used to say that she would forget her head if it wasn't attached. Virginia found, when she was visiting, many of their friends happily made similar jokes about the aging process. Although at the time it seemed that they were merely having a good time, as Virginia thought back on it the humor might have been a defense mechanism. Aging can be frightening. It just happens one day, it doesn't go away, and we don't seem to have much control over it. *Time marches on,* they used to say. *There are only two things in life that are inevitable: death and taxes.* Her parents always had a good sense of humor, even when they were ailing. So did their friends. Laughter seemed to be a good tonic,[11] especially for those all in the same boat, and studies have shown it to be good for the heart and mind.[12]

In those days, Virginia didn't know how to react to this talk since it was so removed from her experience. It would have been impolite to question it so she kept quiet. As a child and well into her adult years, she did not identify with the concept of aging. The lack of elders in her childhood and teen years had left her with no idea of what it is like to lose faculties she had always taken for granted. Watching her parents' ageing was like watching a play from the balcony. The same was true for the disabled, of whom no one ever spoke, and who were generally stared at when seen in public. When she looked back on her younger years, she wondered how she could have missed these things. She had always thought of herself as a considerate person. *How many other people grew up in a similar manner?* The physical problems, the fear, the pain and discomfort were not things in her radar. There is evidence of efforts being made in some communities to integrate the generations, especially youth and elderly, and this will surely be helpful for the future.[13] Virginia's past did not contain this type of input. *It is no wonder,* she thought, *my generation does not know what to do with their elders.* Many people have little experience from which to draw.

Looking back a few generations at her grandparents and beyond, it seemed to Virginia that she had inherited this way of life. The age group who were considered senior citizens in the 1800s is now thought of as relatively young. By 1900, average life expectancy was around forty-seven.[14] Her forefathers had a hard life trying to survive in a new land and the elderly were not strong and often simply did not survive. Although some families, whose children moved around less, managed to stay in the same community and care for the grandparents who lived just down the street, this was not always the case. Grown children, perhaps with families of their own, often had to move where the work was and could not take along *baggage*. So it was with Martin, Virginia's father, who left home at the age of sixteen. He came from a strict upbringing where there was little personal or physical contact with his parents, other than the aforementioned strap when he misbehaved badly. Virginia thought this must explain his attitude toward Grandmother Kress in her later years. His connection with her had always been so remote that he had trouble feeling any compassion for her during her aging process. Perhaps he never thought of it. In spite of his early disconnection with his childhood home, he did recall it from time to time but whenever Virginia asked him to tell her more he would immediately stop talking. Even if the memories of his childhood home were not good, he clearly continued to relate to it as long as his mother still lived in the house.[15] In his and many other cases, the parental home continued to be home until the parents were no longer able to care for themselves. Then the home had to be sold and a new place found for the aging parent. Finding a new home could mean relocating to senior housing or to the home of a family member in another community. In Grandmother Kress's case she *was moved* from the mid-west to California, near Virginia's uncle. The family did not live just down the street.

Reflecting on her parent's situation, Virginia's thoughts drifted to comparing life before her father's retirement to the way it was after that momentous event. Present day society seemed to be as work-oriented as ever and focused on a high tech, fast moving life which lends itself to youth who are eager to stay on the cutting edge. Education is geared toward achievement in the workplace and the rapid changes in technology make it hard to keep up without either diligence and motivation or constant training. She had often heard friends remark they could not figure out something on their computer or on the web. *I'll ask young Alexis,* a ten year old child or grandchild who would know right away what to do. The elastic minds of the younger generation make it easy for them to absorb new methods and they are eager to know all about the latest thing. Their parents pick it up in the workplace because it is a job requirement. Even the top executives now have to know how to type so they can email or send memos. Again, youth wins. [16]

Where does that leave the older generation? Virginia wondered. The elderly often do not have the resources to keep up and find it more difficult to assimilate new ideas. Programming the VCR to record can be a challenge. Her own mother had no idea. How can we carry on a conversation with someone who does not understand megabytes? Some employers consider any information that older workers might have to contribute to be a little fuddy-duddy because their communication skills are so out of date.[17] The lack of employment opportunities can only be discouraging, possibly leading to a diminished sense of self-worth. As people age and become a little more forgetful, what can they contribute? If our elders are unable to contribute to society, does this mean they become a burden? As aging progresses, people slow down. Everything takes longer and youth is impatient. Youth wants and needs fast. The older generation can't cope with this and society shoves them to the side. [18]

However, statistics show that in the United States people over the age of 70 who still work number 1.8 million.[19] Mental skills do not necessarily diminish due to age but processing time does slow down. [20]   Many older workers who have found part-time employment are in a service type position where they can take advantage of flexible schedules. Approximately one third of them are self-employed.[21] Is that because they do not have the financial resources to retire or are they simply bored at the thought? The answer is a little of both and the older people who work are reported to be healthier than those who do not.[22] For sure, as long as they are able to care for themselves, they are not a problem.

What happens when the faculties that we all take for granted start to deteriorate? Seniors become less able-bodied and more dependent on others for things such as shopping, food, bathing and dressing. They are now a problem because they cannot care for themselves and, as such, are in the way of what we think of as progress. As the baby boomers grow older, they will become a large sector of the population requiring some sort of assistance or care.[23] Care can arrive in various settings: home, community or institutional. In any event, it is the family or those responsible for the senior who bears the brunt of the frustration and worry over the well being of their loved one.

Problems arise in a number of ways, whether it is time, other commitments or distance. We still worry and wonder how our senior relative is coping. Virginia sometimes heard people complain that there are not enough hours in the day to hold down a job, take the kids to practice, keep up the yard and visit Grandma. Especially with a young family and a tight schedule, it can be difficult to fit the grandparents in. *We just can't wait for her today. There isn't time to visit.* The grandparents either wait patiently without complaining, not wanting to be a nuisance, or they telephone frequently, demanding one thing or another, or somewhere in between. Virginia's parents were of the first variety. They rarely telephoned; she always called them. They sent birthday cards that they forgot to sign and, occasionally, Christmas presents and they waited for news. They went on about their lives, tucked away with the other *oldsters*. Her mother found some companionship in her church and her father read the paper and seemed to find things to do.

For Virginia, distance was the big problem. When her children were young, they lived many miles from her parents, so she always called them on Sunday afternoon. First, Virginia would talk for a while and then each child would talk. As time went on, her parents had less and less to say. It was difficult to tell if they were not interested in what was going on with her family or if they could not follow the conversation. Eventually, she discovered they both had hearing problems and some of their random comments resulted from the fact that they had misheard what was said. For a while, an amplifier for the phone solved that problem. Virginia found small things like this to be frustrating, often leading to her impatience, even anger. Although a phone conversation cannot compare to actually being there, it can be the next best thing. New technology with video screens so grandparents can see the grandchildren may become a bridge, as long as Grandma can operate the device. Virginia couldn't imagine her mother negotiating a video phone even if it was set up for her and it still does not replace personal contact. [24] Whether Virginia was in the room or on the phone, she generally found herself becoming impatient, not understanding her parents' apparent lack of presence. When she was a child, her mother would tell her to take a deep breath when she felt frustrated about something. She had forgotten that advice when it came to coping with her frustrations with her parents. As it turns out, breathing deeply releases endorphins which calm the nerves, and so her mother's advice, although based on an old wives' tale at the time, was well founded. [25] In a way, the distance made it easier because she could hang up the phone and forget about it until the next time. Later, when her mother lived closer, all the frustrations became amplified.

The real questions are: how did Virginia overcome the difficulty she faced relating to her elders, caring for them and ensuring a reasonable quality of life to help them cope with the aging process? Did she do an adequate job or did she just muddle through? As they aged, how did she stay in touch when they couldn't hear, couldn't move about easily and were increasingly forgetful?

Chapter 2

Cultures

Different cultures in the world view the elders in their population in different ways. Or do they? It could be a difference in environment and circumstance that fosters a different attitude. It could be necessity that files the elders into a category. The definition of that category, in turn, defines the way elders are treated.

When Virginia attended elementary school, the culture in the United States was often referred to as "a melting pot." Her visual imagination had people getting off boats which came from somewhere, being put into a large pot, stirred around with a giant spoon and finally being poured out to find themselves all the same.[26] What bizarre ideas children can come up with! Maybe her idea was understandable however because in her school and community all the people were pretty much the same. There were no African American, Hispanic or Asian children. One time, a boy moved into town from somewhere in the Deep South. He was in her class at school and none of the children could understand his accent. They didn't know how to treat this alien other than to make fun. Now this behavior seems cruel, but at the time, they had no experience with other cultures and didn't know how to react to the unknown. Some would call this a sheltered upbringing. Even summer camp was dirty and dangerous, so Virginia wasn't allowed to go despite her pleas. Until high school, she had no immediate contact with the elderly, sick or disabled or anyone who wasn't just like her.

Virginia's parents did believe in traveling around the country to see memorable sights such as the Liberty Bell, Niagara Falls and the Grand Canyon. The family went to a dude ranch in Arizona where she was allowed to go on trail rides with her father right behind her. Her mother didn't go along very often. She was never one for anything too physical. They also visited antebellum homes in the South. On these trips they always stayed in first class hotels and they, too, all seemed the same. There were never any *different* people in her life.

Finally, when Virginia was in high school, she became a volunteer at the local hospital. This was charitable community service and therefore, acceptable. Other girls were doing it, too. She distributed water bottles to patients' rooms – her first contact with the sick. The uniform was the most exciting part. The one memory that stood out in her mind was entering the darkened room of a dying man and immediately being shooed out by the attending nurse. She found out later it was her friend's father who was dying from cancer. She might have felt bad at the time and she didn't see very much of her friend after his death. This was her first experience with death or near-death. It did not have much of an impact on her life.

It was in her sophomore year of high school that Virginia's parents announced a whirlwind family trip to Europe. The arrangements and deciding exactly what outfit, with matching shoes and purse, would be right for each destination was most exciting. The first stop was Madrid, the beginning of a string of capital cities. The buzz of the fast-moving small cars around the endless squares was exhilarating and the light from old-fashioned lanterns shining in the rivers was romantic to a cloistered teenager. Most of the time on this trip was spent visiting old castles and museums, but there were also occasions when there were glimpses of life in other countries. Of course, they stayed in luxury hotels and rode around in a limousine, but Virginia could look out of the window at passing farms and villages.

Martin had taken up photography in a big way just before the trip, so he was endlessly wandering off looking for photo opportunities. He mainly liked taking pictures of people. He had all types of lenses hanging from his neck and sticking out at a right angle from his torso. Alice did not think much of this posture and would remark about it from time to time. Martin would just grin. Virginia didn't know what to think, so she ignored it. The limo stopped for gas in a dusty village in Spain on the road to Toledo where village elders lounged smoking under a Coca-Cola sign and Martin gave a dollar to an old woman with a goat. Virginia asked him why he had given her money and he said he was paying her for allowing him to take her photograph. That seemed so odd to her at the time but she didn't question it.

In Paris the family visited the Louvre and Notre Dame and were driven up to Sacre Coeur, where Virginia had her portrait painted in the charming square in Montmartre. Artists were everywhere and the scene was so lively and colorful. Oh, how she wanted to stay there and be one of those artists! They seemed so happy with their charcoal and paints. She dreamt about it for months afterward.

In the south of France, they visited a number of villages. The only French Martin knew was *merci beaucoup* so he would walk along the tiny cobbled streets, with his camera dangling, repeating *merci beaucoup* and nodding to all the villagers he met. Alice and Virginia kept their distance. Virginia wore dark glasses and a scarf on her head most of the time. An old woman with a weathered face and no teeth walking slowly up a steep path in a small village attracted Martin's attention with his camera. Shrouded in a long black dress with black socks and sandals and a scarf tied around her head in bandanna fashion only her petite craggy face was visible. She motioned for him to follow her into her narrow house. Martin's broad shoulders turned as he stooped to fit through the slanted doorway. The old woman burst into a toothless smile as she gave everyone strong black French coffee and proudly displayed photographs of her family. Martin was delighted when she allowed him to take her picture. What a wonderful old woman she was. Her home was clean and neat as a pin and the tall rear windows opened up to a beautiful view of the valley. Virginia wondered why she had to travel all that way to meet this old lady when plenty like her must have been waiting at home.

In spite of the limousines, this trip was Virginia's first eye-opener to the idea of cultural differences. The melting pot suddenly acquired a history and from then on she wanted nothing more than to travel and meet people who were different from those she had known at home. College represented the great escape because, although it was a small private girls' college, it was a thousand miles away from Chicago. Although she did not cut herself off from her parents and she called them every week, she never went back to their home to live. She studied a foreign language and after college moved to Europe where she remained for over twenty years.

In Europe and other parts of the world, Virginia had observed elders treated with respect. In Great Britain, where she spent the majority of her time, people her age were always off to visit grandparents who usually seemed to be in the country or at the seaside. The families she knew seemed to include all the generations in outings or family events. Entire families would show up at the pub, especially at Sunday lunch, the men standing at the bar with a pint and the ladies taking a seat. It was common to see a grandparent at school events and certainly at holidays. The Queen Mum, the eldest of the royal family, was everyone's favorite.

During the years Virginia spent living in Britain, her new family, husband and two daughters, traveled across the Channel to the Continent. They skied in the Alps, visited major cities and spent summer holidays on the Mediterranean coast. In southern Europe, elderly ladies were a part of the local scene as they banded together in small groups, usually dressed in black. They could be seen sitting in front of a house or on park benches while the children played nearby. They could be seen at church, at the market, at cafes, or teahouses. They were part of the family and the community, not shut away in retirement complexes where no one ever saw them. All of the elderly people appeared to be healthy and able to move around and care for themselves. None of them needed full time care or nursing. As far as Virginia knew, the family took in the elderly when they could not cope on their own. In many cases, all generations continued to live under the same roof and there were usually neighbors who had become firm friends available to help if needed.

The culture shock Virginia had experienced living abroad was not enormous. The European heritage of the United States was evident in many religious and social customs. When she moved back to the States, she landed on the west coast, in California, but the travel bug had settled in her heart and her eyes were drawn west, across the Pacific. On her first trip, she visited the beautiful rugged country of Nepal. Sandwiched between India and China and nestled in the shadows of the giant Himalayas, it was, at the time, considered to be the poorest country in the world. She was excited to visit the capital city, Katmandu, remembering the romantic name from Aunt Rose. It was a very busy place with lots of small, stinky vehicles whizzing around, people very determined to get somewhere soon, other people determined to sell you something you don't want, cows standing around or meandering down the street, dogs looking for something to eat - all of this going on in narrow dusty cobbled streets with open sewers along the sides. In Thamel, the tourist section, there were orderly shops, restaurants, an Internet café - which made communication possible except when the satellite went behind the mountains - and plenty of street vendors selling everything imaginable. Sometimes, young men would follow her down the street encouraging her to buy a few beads. A disabled man begged on a corner and a young woman clutching a disfigured child held out her hand. In other parts of the city, especially in the busy market section, the elderly sat in front of what must have been the family shop.

Religion is an important part of the culture in Nepal. There are many temples and shrines both in the cities and in the countryside. Nepal is a mixture of Hindu and Buddhist religions which exist harmoniously together, each respecting the traditions of the other. During the week of an important religious festival, Virginia and her younger daughter, Charlotte, were staying in a smaller city some distance from Katmandu. A small shrine was situated just outside their shuttered hotel window and all day people came to pray, offer a sacrifice and afterward, ring the gong. A few sleepless nights ensued because they continued to come to pray all night, each time ringing the gong. The prayers were often giving thanks for food or in connection with the health of a family member.

Traveling through the countryside of Nepal, Virginia and Charlotte were struck by the beauty of the rugged scenery. The people were wonderful and inventive farmers and they turned the mountainside into picturesque terraces with an array of crops. Most of the rural roads were impassable, other than by foot, so everything was carried by people or animals. The terraces were too narrow and steep for farming equipment so planting was done by hand or with the help of animals. Outside a small village, a young father was teaching his son how to plant a field with an ox-drawn plough. The boy had the long leather strap, which was attached to the head of the ox to serve as reins, tied around his waist. Holding a wooden plough in both hands like a giant wishbone, he struggled to push it behind the ox through the heavy soil. It was difficult because the ox was not particularly interested in this activity but father and son received plenty of advice from a group of old men who sat along a wall at the edge of the small field. As Virginia and Charlotte left this project, they passed by one of many round earth huts along the climbing path and the young woman standing in front of the single small opening invited them inside. It was dark, lit only by the fire. The smoke, some of which did not escape through the hole in the roof, invaded the small room. When their eyes adjusted, they found an old woman lying on a blanket and a small child playing on the dirt floor. Virginia felt drawn by a warm family atmosphere and it became apparent that all generations lived together in this hut.

A few years after her trip to Asia an opportunity arose for Virginia to visit Peru and she jumped at it. Many miles from the giant Himalayas, Lima is a modern city but her group traveled inland to Cusco.[27] The altitude in the Andes rivaled her trek in Nepal near Annapurna[28] and one member of her small party became very ill. The local hotels were used to tourists with altitude sickness and bustled around with oxygen tanks. In the countryside the terrain was steep but the soil is rich and the terraced farming was reminiscent of Nepal. Many hikers choose to follow the Inca Trail to reach Machu Picchu, the ancient Inca sanctuary, but Virginia's group took the train which slowly snaked through the scenic mountains emerging through the fog at its destination. She found Machu Picchu to be a spiritual place which was most evident at daybreak when the first sunbeams sliced through the atmosphere and cast long shadows in the temple. As she stood on the ridge facing east, trekkers emerged from the Trail behind her just in time to catch the breaking light.

Traveling through Peru on a small coach or by train, she had an opportunity to observe villages and lifestyle. The Catholic Church is strong in many parts of South America and there were churches as well as small shrines for the traveler along the road. In the villages, the elderly were found in small groups, dressed in all black as in southern Europe. One old woman was very upset when some of the party tried to take her picture. Thinking the camera would capture her spirit, she started throwing things to chase the invaders away. Virginia's group was invited into a musty dark hut which turned out to be the village hang-out and pub. Only men were inside but they were of all ages. An old shrunken man stirred a brown liquid in a barrel. He was the master who beckoned them forward to try some of the strong local brew.

Only last year, Virginia was lucky enough to be able to go on a trip to China, a country she had never before visited. The party flew to Shanghai and traveled from there into the interior of the country. They were a small group of eleven and everyone, except Virginia, was a photographer, some amateur and some professional. A great variety of equipment, lenses, bodies, tripods and filters were carried, dragged, pulled and pushed across fields, up hills, down hills, and along narrow paths. A tremendous amount of time was spent setting up cameras, focusing, moving two feet, refocusing, and waiting for the shot. Virginia had prudently brought along her smallest point-and-shoot digital camera so she had none of these problems. She used her wait time to observe the surroundings, the structures and mostly the people. They were all shapes, sizes and ages. The elderly could often be found sitting on a chair or stoop watching and waiting. Sometimes, they were inside a shop, with an open door, watching TV. She was instantly reminded of rural Peru, Nepal and so many other places.

On the trip, the guide in Shanghai, Andie, reported that care facilities for the elderly in Shanghai are on the rise. Andie's uncle, much to her mother's dismay, had installed her grandmother in one such facility. Andie was unhappy with the situation, but apparently, there was nothing she could do. Her uncle had the final say. Andie made it quite clear nursing homes did not represent the traditional way of caring for the family elders. As in Nepal and Peru, the elders would have remained in the home, cared for by the family members. However, China is undergoing rapid and dramatic economic and social change. The changes in Chinese way of life, which mimics our own, include the introduction of long-term care. Virginia wondered how this development will affect the family structure.

One thing that became clear to Virginia during these glimpses into other cultures was the similarity in their approach to life. Families remained together and the sick and elderly were cared for within the family unit.[29] This could have been due to necessity arising out of meager means, but the traditional view of life seemed to be holistic, incorporating body, mind and spirit as a unit and the unit included family. It also included a God or Creator as the anchor of the belief system. Rituals and ceremonies played an important part in family and in society. Ill health was thought to arise out of a need for the higher consciousness to communicate with the "personality consciousness".[30] It raised the level of awareness of life. The earth, the land and its provisions were not taken for granted, but considered to be an integral part of life.[31] Aging and death were valued and honored as a part of life's journey.

During her time in Europe, Virginia became and accomplished artist, a love she thought she had inherited from her father. After he and her mother moved to Florida he had spent many hours painting beach scenes and decorating pieces of driftwood. Perhaps it was an outgrowth of his years in the advertising industry and in retirement he finally had time to pursue his talent. A few years before her trip to China, Virginia was asked to do a painting of a Native American chief. To gather research information for her image she attended pow-wows. On one particular occasion, the celebration took place in a park in the heart of a large city. All ages were present, the youngest in strollers and the oldest sitting in chairs around the edge of a large circle with a fire smoldering in the center. Men, women and children danced around the circle, intent on the beat of the music. Sitting on the edge she observed the colorful costumes and listened to the drums beating from inside a tent. Suddenly there was silence and everyone returned to the edge. An elderly man proudly wearing a magnificent white headdress advanced into the circle and announced the celebration that day was in memory of Oscar, an elder who had recently passed away.

Family members had made long journeys from many parts of the country to pay tribute. Several of them took turns speaking about Oscar, recalling his life with fond memories. Toward the end, Virginia wished she had known him. The drums started again and nearly everyone rose and joined in the dancing, making small steps in time to the music. The younger members supported the elderly so they could dance as well. Someone beckoned her to join in the dancing which she did, stepping to the beat in memory of Oscar.

The pow-wows sparked a curiosity in Virginia to learn more about Native American traditions which turned out to be a good example of the holistic view of life. Everything in life is connected, creating "one".[32]   Nature and animals are "respected and protected" because they contribute to the collective harmony of the world.[33] The spirit is of utmost importance and the body is "the earthly robe" or manifestation of the spirit. Through the body, the spirit can interpret life on earth. Healers (shamans) use spiritual energy to effect healing of the earthly body. The shaman is often a tribal elder who has been through a long training period.[34] He or she is a person held apart from the rest of the tribe because a spiritual connection gives him, or her, the vision to help others.[35] Miracle healings, occurring though tribal rituals, are often not accepted by the patient's doctors. Medical doctors prefer to call such healings a misdiagnosis.[36]

Ceremonies are powerful. The beating of the drums, the smoke from the fire and the dancing are all hypnotic means of reaching the higher consciousness of the spiritual world. Not only does a ceremony help the spirit on its journey, but it can also facilitate healing of the body by returning it to a balanced state.[37]   Some Native Americans have moved away from the ancient ways in preference to western culture. However, the shamans live on with pride.

With individual cultural heritages in the limelight and some traditions even revived, the question is: how will the elders fare? Immigrant families in the United States tend to cling to traditional cultural values. Many have come from poor circumstances in their native countries where they were unable to seek medical care and instead they used traditional alternative healing methods. Their situations remain similar when they come to the United States. They are suspicious of establishment systems and are not comfortable divulging personal information to strangers. Latino family values which include respect for elders, personal connections, spirituality and the role of destiny remain strong. This group tends to avoid hospitals.[38] Immigrant Afghan families bring with them cultural values which include the feeling that they must do everything possible for elders.[39] In Asian families there is usually a spokesperson who has taken on the role of decision maker for family health issues. Often there is rivalry among siblings. So far the increasing higher education of younger generations has not diminished the value of the decision maker role.[40] However there is evidence of a shift away from multi-generational households in Latino families[41] and second and third generation Asian families move to the suburbs to rear their children. In later generations cultural family values therefore become dissipated.[42] Will traditional family care ultimately be thrown into the melting pot only to reappear in the shape of institutions for the sake of convenience?

Chapter 3

The Looks of Aging

Why is it that the elderly become so inconvenient and difficult to care for that we no longer want them at home? Growing up as Virginia did, without many older people around, she did not have much comprehension of the effects of aging and the changes she saw in her parents prompted some questions. What seems to happen to the body and mind as the years pass? As a younger person, she didn't even wonder. Watching her aunt and her parents decline in function she saw their need for assistance increase. Aunt Rose slowed down from her tremendous pace and went from traveling the world to being content to stay in her apartment in Florida. She had always possessed a remarkable curiosity about everything, but as her years increased her energy declined diminishing the level of interest. She did however have a great sense of humor and it stayed with her until she died. Although Virginia was close to her aunt, she had never spent extended periods of time with her and changes in her behavior were not a concern. When Virginia saw her in her later years, she did notice that her aunt seemed to tire quickly, spending a lot of time sleeping. Her mother would comment on it from time to time.

Virginia's parents kept up their activities but she couldn't help noticing a change in their level of interest and energy. They were always on the go but suddenly, they, like her aunt, became content to stay at home. One year, they went on a family vacation to Sedona, Arizona. Alice hadn't been to that area in many years but Virginia remembered from her childhood how her parents loved the southwest. She was confident they would enjoy the trip. The blooming desert flowers were exquisite and the contrast between the red rocks and blue sky was straight out of a travel magazine. The day after their arrival Alice started asking when they would be leaving. No amount of scenery, excursions, entertainment or shopping could distract her from her goal. *When were they going home?* On the morning when they were set to leave, around mid-day, the children were enjoying a last swim in the hotel pool. Virginia found her mother sitting on the edge of her bed, dressed for the trip with suitcase packed and firmly closed. Virginia was disappointed at the outcome of this vacation and learned a lesson. No more trips. Her mother seemed to have lost the spirit of adventure that she had inherited. At the time, she didn't understand the meaning of this type of behavior. She was used to both of her parents being more active, eager to explore and see new things. She didn't want a change in the status quo. She easily grew impatient with them and reacted by leaving to go back to her own life and, although she still worried, she wasn't sure what she was worrying about. As her parents were aging, they were changing before her eyes.

At the time of the Sedona trip, although her parents did not have specific physical limitations other than a little stiffness and moving more slowly, they did not like being out of their comfort zone. Unfamiliar territory away from home made them anxious and insecure. What if they got sick? The doctor was a long way away. Virginia discovered that environment, especially familiar surroundings, plays a large part in the sense of well-being. This was even more obvious with Aunt Rose whose home was important and gave her confidence. In her eighties, her aunt moved out of her house and into an apartment in Florida. No one forced her. It was her choice. The apartment was stuffed with collectible artifacts and furniture she had acquired from around the world. She had finally given up traveling except for one visit, when she was eighty-three, to Singapore, her favorite city and one she knew well. She knew it would be her last trip so she stayed for several months. When Virginia went to visit her parents, Martin would pick up Aunt Rose and bring her down to stay for a few days. As Aunt Rose grew older, Virginia noticed that she was a little unsteady on her feet and seemed a bit confused during these short visits. She would apologize for walking slowly. The minute she returned to her apartment she was fine again. She became confident and happy to be hostess when she was in her own environment, surrounded by familiar things. She felt secure in her new building: she played bridge with fellow residents, had a cocktail before dinner, and was generally happy. The relationship between aging and environment seems to be a close one. Familiarity breeds confidence and fosters independence. In Aunt Rose's case, the aging process seemed to be gradual and graceful, especially with a little assistance.[43] She remained independent until, at the age of ninety, she passed away peacefully. That is not the case with everyone.

A serious illness can have an especially devastating effect, not only on the sick person, but also on the family. The person is suddenly in need of constant care and attention which can include doctors' visits, hospital visits, medication and help with their daily routine. Chronic illness can ultimately lead to physical disability and increased dependence. Of those older adults living in some level of residential care facility, around 80% are suffering from some form of continuing disability.[44] Virginia began to recognize that some sort of trauma, such as a serious illness or the death of a loved one, can quickly accelerate the aging process, not only of the ailing person, but also of the family members. As long as her aunt was alive, her mother was always the young one. As soon as her elder sister passed away, her mother began to show her age. She seemed to age in spurts. She would be the same for maybe a year or more and then, suddenly, she was older. These spurts, part of the normal aging process, could also have been manifestations of the reaction to the grief from the loss of her sister.[45]

Virginia's father changed dramatically in a short time due to illness. Since Virginia had never had much to do with the gravely ill or dying, she didn't know what to expect when he told her he had *come down with a nasty case of lung cancer,* as her put it in an attempt to belittle the disease. In the middle of the summer she arrived at a steamy Jacksonville airport and took a cab to their apartment in the retirement complex. Her mother came to the door and ushered her in. Martin was sitting in a chair by the window and did not immediately get up. She was stunned when she saw him. From the tall, robust and upright man that she had always known and had seen a few months prior, he had lost about sixty pounds, was frail and stooped with a grayish complexion and using an oxygen mask. A shocking transformation! Virginia was unprepared. She took herself off to the hairdresser to mull it over. She found it hard to be in the house with him trailing his oxygen tank around as a constant reminder of his illness. She did not realize at the time how hard it was on her mother who was dedicated to his doctors' appointments, his tests and driving him back and forth. It was kind of a role reversal because Martin had never allowed anyone to drive but him and now he couldn't provide this manly service. Alice, being of short stature, hardly seeing over the steering wheel, was not a good driver. She knew it. She would refuse to drive the grandchildren anywhere. Martin was in the position of being driven by her. He hated it. Still, he retained his sense of humor and optimism joking about Alice's driving. They went out for dinner to the nearby country club overlooking the Atlantic. Martin hardly touched the lobster tail, one of his favorites. Virginia could see he was failing rapidly.

Virginia returned to her family but was recalled about four months later to her father's bedside. This time he was dying. He wasn't ready to give up though and he lingered for a few weeks in the hospital with pneumonia. She and her mother visited daily. She felt terrible, but she couldn't bring herself to touch him. She didn't know if she was afraid that she might catch something or not; it was just something she couldn't do. She would stand away from the bed or sit in the chair. She noticed her mother didn't want to touch him either. They were never a touchy, huggy family and this time was no exception. Thinking back on that time, Virginia wondered if it would have made a difference to him if they had just held his hand.

She felt a strange sense of helplessness. The doctors were resigned and said they could not help her father and it was just a matter of time. He couldn't speak because the cancer had moved into his throat. He was frustrated at not being able to communicate; he had always been a great talker. Virginia made a card with the alphabet on it in the hope he could spell out what he wanted to say, but he just didn't have the strength. She was disappointed. He went into a coma in the last few days. Though he appeared to be unconscious, Virginia was sure that he could still hear them talking. The doctors seemed to know, too. They always stepped out of the room to talk about his condition.

It was strange seeing him dead. She had never seen a dead person before. He didn't look very different and she wondered where he had gone. In a way she felt relieved when he finally died; it was so hard seeing him that way. He had always been so tall and strong and this disease had crushed him like an ant. Virginia's husband and children came for the funeral. It was kind of like a party, but it felt incomplete because her father wasn't there. Her mother said she couldn't believe he wouldn't come walking in the door. It took some time for Alice to accept the reality of his death. She seemed smaller and a little helpless without him. The grieving process can take some time and it was hard for Virginia to tell when her mother stopped grieving.[46]

People react differently to loss. An elderly couple had lived next door to Virginia's parents and whenever she and the children came to visit the wife brought over desserts. She didn't go out much and spent her time consumed with a hobby of making jewelry, lots of little glittering animal brooches and necklaces which she insisted on giving the children. One day her husband died suddenly on the golf course and his mousy wife of fifty-some years went right out and bought a convertible car and a red hat. She became quite the gad-about-town. Virginia's mother also had been a fairly solitary person who liked to read and spend time by herself. After her husband's death, she continued to live in their apartment in the retirement community and Virginia still lived a good distance away. She hadn't made many new friends there because she and Martin had been so consumed with his health that there had been little time for anything else. Martin had always been the social one, and he hadn't felt much like socializing when he was ill. Unlike her neighbor, now Alice spent even more time by herself and became more introverted. She even seemed to give up her involvement with the church. Virginia was surprised at this sudden lack of interest because church activities had always been a big part of her life. The American Geriatrics Society reports that "religious involvement" and good health seem to go hand-in-hand. It provides a like-minded, non-judgmental social group and appears to be helpful to the aging process.[47]   Alice suddenly dropped it. Virginia wondered why at the time but Alice came up with some excuse like she didn't know anyone any more.

Alice did not go to the dining room for dinner because she said there was a stigma attached to eating alone. Reasonable, Virginia thought, because she would not want to go to eat alone either, although many people do. The real insight here would have been to understand her mother's sense of loss of her way of life. Life wasn't the same without Martin. Coming from a generation where the man was the provider and needed to do everything, she had relied on him for many years. She didn't know how to go out by herself and she felt it was too late or too much effort to learn. Furthermore, during his illness she had been his caregiver and that had become her whole world.   Now, not only had she lost him, but she had lost her reason for being.[48] Withdrawal from activities and life in general can be a manifestation of grief.[49] For Alice the grief was not only for loss of her husband but also loss of her lifestyle. Virginia was unaware of this at the time and, living far away, she didn't know how to monitor her mother's activities.

Loss of a life partner is considered to be a major life event. Grief typically lasts six to twelve months,[50] but it can spiral out of control. Thinking back on her mother's behavior, Virginia wondered how much lifestyle plays a part in the amount of grief suffered. *Can grief even be measured? How do you know how I feel?* In her parents' generation, when the little woman stayed at home and kept the house, the partner was everything so the loss was overwhelming. Today, we see many two-income families and each partner has a life outside the marriage. However work or busyness cannot make up for the loss of a life partner; the effects are just as overwhelming and grief just as intense. "Actress Helen Hayes, describing the two years following her husband's death, has these devastating words to say: 'I was just as crazy as you can be and still be at large. I didn't have any really normal minutes during those years. It wasn't just grief. It was total confusion.'"[51] Confusion would have been a good word to describe Virginia's mother. She went from being organized, even controlling, to being unable to complete a task that had been important to her in the past. At first Virginia was not worried and thought her mother would adjust. Grief can manifest in many ways, ranging from denial to confusion, from sadness to fear and many things in between. There can also be physical symptoms such as shortness of breath. The grief-stricken can become forgetful, disorganized and irritable. They can suffer from insomnia and loss of appetite. All of these applied to Alice.[52]

Fairly soon after Martin's death Virginia and the children came for a visit during a school holiday. They rented a condominium near the beach and not far from Alice's complex. Arriving at Alice's apartment, Virginia found her mother was already getting to the stage where she didn't seem to notice things like the mail piling up or rotten food in the refrigerator. She wasn't sure what to do about it since she could not oversee these things on a daily basis. At first, she tried talking to her mother in the hope she would pay more attention. Soon it became apparent that this tactic was not working. Alice was beginning to find daily activities overwhelming, so she didn't do them.

It was on that visit that they had arranged to meet Alice at the country club for lunch. By this time she had been living in the area for a few years. She still had her car and drove to the store so Virginia was not concerned about her driving herself to the restaurant. Virginia and the children arrived first and waited for half an hour or so after which she started calling the apartment. After the third call, Alice answered. Virginia asked if she remembered she was supposed to meet them and Alice replied that she had become lost so she went back home. This was her neighborhood. It wasn't a large city, only a small resort town. *She got lost?* This was the first episode.

Virginia and the children returned home and continued to call regularly. She always asked her mother what she had had for lunch or dinner the night before. Often the answer was a hard-boiled egg or a piece of toast. At least she didn't lie. Food preparation was another one of those daily tasks she seemed to have let fall by the wayside and she refused to go to the dining room for dinner. Virginia started wondering about nutrition and her overall health.

At times during their regular calls, Alice had difficulty following the conversation and would come out with unrelated remarks. Talking to her on the phone became increasingly difficult. At one stage, Virginia decided to have her mother's hearing tested again and it turned out her hearing had deteriorated even further to where she could hardly hear anything out of one ear and about 50% out of the other. Virginia knew her parents both had hearing problems.

Alice would accuse Martin of speaking softly and he would counter with her mumbling. She was not, however, aware that her mother's hearing was that bad because she had become quite clever about hiding it. No wonder she couldn't carry on a conversation; she didn't know what was being said. "Sensory limitations, especially hearing and vision loss, also increase with advanced age. . . Both of these sensory deficits are significantly associated with functional decline."[53]   New hearing aids helped until Virginia discovered that her mother wasn't wearing them. She had misplaced them she said. *They really haven't been perfected yet. They buzz. They are uncomfortable.* All kinds of excuses! Alice wasn't interested in what people were saying anyway. Virginia started to grow impatient with that attitude. *Was my reaction unusual?* Virginia wondered. Many people feel the same way.[54]

On the next visit to her mother, when Virginia planned to stay longer, she found the desk again piled high with unopened mail and papers. As she began to go through it she found checks, some for substantial amounts, which had not been deposited. Alice had always been on top of her financial situation and this really was a cause for concern. This incident provoked Virginia to hire a local conservator who would oversee all the bills and arrange for a staff person to come in regularly to check on her mother. She thought the facility should have been doing that, but it was a newly built place and they were not up to speed on everything. Maybe that was not even part of their job. She wasn't sure, so she solved the problem herself at least temporarily or so she thought. As it turned out, her mother did not take kindly to the person who came to look in on her. Virginia began to get reports that Alice wouldn't open the door or stay in the same room with the kindly lady. As far as she was concerned, the woman was uninvited and she resented this invasion into her privacy.

Feeling needed at home by her own children, one of who required extra attention, Virginia was on a short fuse when it came to her mother. It seemed as though Alice had become another child for whom she had to care. Judith Viorst says in *Necessary Losses:*

> "As our parents succumb to the frailties of the flesh, their needs encroach on our time and our equanimity. We're caught up again in their lives and there is much talk of money and health on the telephone. Our children, now grown, can take care of themselves, but can a widowed mother or father live alone? With impatience, resentment, sorrow and guilt accompanying, and at times outweighing, our love, we physically and emotionally accommodate to our parents' growing dependencies. In mid-life we discover that we are destined to become our parents' parents. Few of us factored this into our life's plan."[55]

Those in middle age are sometimes referred to as the *sandwich generation* because we have responsibility for the generations on either side – our children and our parents. This is a hard place to be. Strings are pulling in both directions and the question of who is most important often comes up.

Enlisting the help of trained professionals can lift the burden of the parent generation. However, for Virginia, it did not come without a price – guilt. Inevitably, it seemed, she worried if her mother was being cared for properly. Should she be doing this at home? Yes, the majority of long-term care is given at home and most often, by family members. The government has eased the financial burden by allowing family caregivers to be paid,[56] but for some of us, it is impossible to integrate a needy elder into our lives. Must we make a choice? Virginia considered the difference between caring for the young, who are looking forward to life, and caring for the older generation, who are thinking of death. The one is always more appealing and the other more depressing. *The choice is easy,* she rationalized; the children need us. We are after all a "child-orientated society"[57] because children are the breath of the future. *Not so fast,* she thought; our elders need us, too – just in a different way. What, then, do they have to offer? Not youth, high energy and expanding minds. Instead, they have a quiet wisdom and much life experience to give. Remembering the enthusiasm of Aunt Rose as she told tales of her history, Virginia envisioned her mother's experiences clinging to her. Seniors want to share. It is a kind of validation that their lives have been witnessed. Partners are generally considered witnesses, but if one dies there is a void. Sharing enhances the quality of life and improves overall health and seniors particularly love to tell stories;[58] Alice certainly did. Communication is a key factor, even for those who have lost verbal abilities, but communicating with her mother was becoming difficult.

Sitting in her mother's apartment one afternoon listening to the thunder and waiting for the inevitable rain to start drumming on the roof, Virginia continued to ponder her mother's aging, something that she had not accurately addressed. After all, she was not exactly getting younger. *Aging is a curious process,* she thought. Maybe it's not so curious when it's happening to you or someone close to you. When it is happening to you, it suddenly becomes very personal. Instead of: *Oh, look at that poor person in a wheel chair,* it is you in the wheel chair, looking up at the world from a different viewpoint. So what does aging do to us? She realized that she didn't have a clear idea.

Some years later, in an internet search, Virginia found The American Society on Aging which comments on their web site that: "As we grow older, it often becomes difficult to use many everyday products because of arthritis and other conditions."[59] Difficulty using some products was another way of saying that aging restricts options and control of lifestyle. The usual way of doing things becomes difficult and we have to adapt. Changes can be difficult for anyone, more so for those who have been used to doing everyday activities the same way for years, such as putting on a sweater or brushing their teeth. That is just the beginning. Virginia tried to imagine, as she sat typing on her laptop, that the time might soon come when she would have difficulty typing anything. Not only could it be problematic moving her fingers, but it could also be difficult for her brain to connect the appropriate keys to the letters of the words that she wanted to communicate. Maybe she wouldn't even know what she wanted to communicate! That was a scary thought and, in some cases, it seemed to be an understatement.

Other conditions, Virginia thought, could be anything from stiff fingers due to arthritis, to using a walker or wheel chair due to a broken hip, paralysis due to an accident or stroke, mental confusion and disorganization due to dementia, just to name a few. Often, older people get along just fine by themselves. She revisited the situation of her aunt compared to her mother. Familiar surroundings and routine increases confidence and along with that comes independence and security. [60]   Virginia remembered that her aunt was much more confident in her own surroundings than when she was in an unfamiliar place. She knew her way around her apartment and where everything was kept. She knew her building and the local shops. She had her walker or cane to help with her balance. She lived alone until she was ninety and was able to care for herself. She had no cognitive problems. Alice was a different story. Alice had always been less independent than her sister and became forgetful and confused even in her own town. She needed more assistance, perhaps supervision which meant loss of independence. The American Society of Aging offered suggestions on their web site of in-home organizing items that can help seniors remain independent.[61]

When function becomes severely compromised in later life, this decline can turn into chronic disability. Quite suddenly, there is a huge change in lifestyle forced on us. We don't choose it; it simply happens one day. Going from walking around to using a wheel chair is a big production. Unless you are lucky enough to have an electric wheel chair, you must have a lot of upper body strength to move yourself around. Going in and out of doors becomes an obstacle. What if there is a step or a hill? Up or down, it can be dangerous. The other option is to rely on someone to push you around, move you in and out of the chair, take you to the toilet, etc. Independence is gone. Loss of function can be overwhelming and can trigger the same type of grief reaction as if a loved one had died. Family members often do not recognize what is actually happening.[62] As the boomers age, more and more people will have this disposition. Many elderly do suffer from some sort of chronic disability and daily tasks become difficult, if not outright dangerous.

This situation raises the issue of long-term care. When aging problems necessitate some type of care, it can be a relative, friend, community service or paid care providing assistance. The majority of care comes from family members, but varying levels of community based, assisted living and nursing home care have been increasing.[63] Although the percentage of older adults suffering from chronic disability is actually declining, the real numbers are increasing due to the increase in the size of the older population.[64] The boomers are reaching that age and many of them are living longer. By the year 2020, it is estimated that 14 million persons in the United States will need long-term care.[65] With Alzheimer's patients alone, it is believed the numbers will grow considerably. The baby boomers have benefited from better education and better nourishment than the preceding generation and that means their life expectancy with the disease will double. The nursing home stay for an Alzheimer's patient is approximately twice that of others.[66] Virginia's thoughts shifted from her mother to herself. She could see old age before her and wondered what can be done to ease the burden that the population change will produce.

The expression "quality of life" comes up often in relation to seniors and the disabled and it raises a number of questions. What does it mean? Who decides what is *good quality of life* and what isn't? What are the signs indicating a deteriorating quality of life for seniors? When should one intervene and who should intervene? How are we to cope with this problem? At what stage do we have to take charge in order to ensure safety and at least a consistent quality of life?

The Quality of Life Research Unit at the University of Toronto has put quality of life for seniors neatly into three categories. The first category is being: physical being (getting around, eating the right foods), psychological being (clear thoughts, coping with life) and spiritual being (a sense of accomplishment, participation in spiritual activities). The second category is called belonging: physical belonging (privacy, adaptation for seniors if necessary), social belonging (family members and neighbors on whom to rely) and community belonging (getting health services, going places in the neighborhood). The third category is becoming: practical becoming (caring for another person, doing chores around the home), leisure becoming (hobbies, recreational activities), and growth becoming (mental acuity, adjusting to changes in life).[67] To sum up, it comes down to a sense of well-being and control of one's life on a personal and social basis. Presumably then, if one or more of these categories slips out of control, quality of life also slips a bit, and maybe then a bit more. At what point do we determine that enough slippage is enough and the person is in need of help?

When talking with care managers one often hears references to "Activities of Daily Living (ADL)" and "Instrumental Activities of Daily Living (IADL)"[68] in relation to seniors. ADLs include basic living activities such as bathing, dressing, eating, toileting, and grooming. When one or more of these functions is compromised there is cause for concern. IADLs are deemed to be less critical. They include activities such as housework, shopping and laundry.[69] The ability to move around comes under a separate category. Strategies to help anyone with a functional decline have been defined.[70] Safety for the loved one seems to be a common theme. Ultimately, with advice from the medical practitioner involved, the decision to intervene seems to be up to the family member or responsible party.

A problem can arise when the older person in need of help refuses to accept it. When Virginia was away in college, her mother told her on the phone that her father had to fly out to get Grandmother Kress out of her house. *What for?* Virginia asked. Apparently, it was decided that she could no longer care for herself and should be moved to a nursing home. Alarmed at the thought, she had locked herself in the house refusing all comers, even Uncle Eddy. Martin must have convinced her she couldn't stay there by herself because she did move into the nursing home near Uncle Eddy. Virginia was disinterested at the time and went on to tell her mother about some class she was taking, but the memory stayed with her.

All of this information was news to Virginia. During the time when she was worrying about her mother, she did not have access to resources that might help her nor time to look for them. Virginia started to see her mother's difficulties as signs that she needed some supervision to ensure her safety and health. No more getting lost! It was time to act. Enter the long-term care facility.

Chapter 4

Moving Mother

About thirty years ago, Philip Slater in *Pursuit of Loneliness* identified a tendency in our society that he called the "Toilet Assumption." The idea is that anything problematic, such as people who are difficult to deal with, vanishes if it is merely "removed from our immediate field of vision." The remedy for the elderly, mentally challenged or infirm is to place them in an institution where we don't have to think about them. If, down the line, they come to our attention again, we are *shocked* and immediately take steps to ensure they safely disappear again.[71] It may be that the situation has not changed much since Slater's day. What happens to people when they disappear into *the home?* Virginia's parents, especially her mother, went through various stages of senior living accommodations.

At the retirement community level, residents are very active, at least these days. Seniors seem to be happy not to have annoying young families around and eagerly embrace the activities provided to keep them occupied. From the outside, these communities appear to be quite normal and life goes on with the newspaper and the mail arriving at the door, people going out for coffee or playing golf and tennis. No one is locked in. People come and go as they always have. When Martin was so ill, Alice had moved him and herself into their first community in Florida which provided all levels of care, from independent living right up to skilled nursing, should it be required.

The state of Florida seems to attract people of retirement age for several reasons. One obvious reason is the climate. Although the temperature varies, there is not the extreme weather of the northern states. It seems as though Florida is home to more elderly people than any other state in the USA and a large older population has fostered amenities for that age group. There are also facilities offering a higher level of care. With an older population increase in other states, these types of facilities have spread, but at the time of Virginia's parents' retirement, they were not prevalent.

This community worked out fine for Martin when he was ill because his wife was on the spot to make sure he received the appropriate care. When it came to Alice, things were a little different. No one was looking in on her on a regular basis to make sure she was all right. The facility was new and untested as far as the organization was concerned. That is not to say they were doing a bad job but small things overlooked can have a big impact.

The assisted living level is another type of community where the residents socialize but may need help with bathing and food preparation. This is the fastest growing sector of senior living facilities.[72] The American Society on Aging describes them like this: "Most assisted living facilities offer personalized care and support services, including meals served in a common dining area or taken to a resident's room, shuttles for errands and appointments, housekeeping, help with medication management and emergency call monitoring. Assisted living facilities also offer some resident supervision."[73] Alice's second apartment in Florida was in this category. Her apartment was very nice, and Virginia had it redecorated to her taste and made some alterations to accommodate her furniture. She had a parking space for her car, but Virginia soon discovered that she didn't go out much. Although she had her own kitchen, there was also a pleasant dining room where meals were provided or a tray could be brought to the apartment. Alice usually opted for this latter service since she didn't like eating alone and didn't know many people whom she could join in the dining room.

The final stage is the skilled nursing facility which is where Virginia mysteriously found herself working. Her experience with her mother in a care facility had been slightly hit or miss. In the early 1900s, some states decided to place regulatory controls on the development of nursing homes. This decision resulted in a skewed supply and demand in many areas.[74] Growth of nursing homes has been restricted in states requiring a certificate of need and, considering the probability of needing nursing home care is about 49% by the age of 85, government policies come under scrutiny.[75] Despite that fact, many seniors think they will never have a need for nursing home care.[76]

At first, it is disturbing to realize that these people are here waiting to die. As long as the money holds out, they will never live anywhere else. Many of these facilities offer Alzheimer's care and these units are usually locked so the residents don't wander off and get lost. Nursing homes must comply with Federal regulations in order to participate in Medicare and Medicaid programs;[77] they are regularly inspected. The American Society on Aging offers this advice: "Reliable nursing home ratings can help you find the best nursing home for your loved one. Your choice of a nursing home could have a profound impact on their quality of life and sense of dignity. But, which nursing home is best? Are some nursing homes better than others? Several services have compiled nursing home ratings to help answer both questions."[78] They also offer lists of counselors and other professionals who can advise on choosing a facility, and they include a checklist on how to pay for it.[79] In some communities there are more choices than in others. Understanding that the choice of facility has such an "impact on quality of life and sense of dignity" really hit home for Virginia. Whereas in the community at large, senior centers and facilities create a support structure that can have a positive influence on health and quality of life, the nursing care facility is a closed environment. The facility itself becomes a new community for the residents and the sense of community can have either a positive or negative effect on health. A positive environment can be life sustaining and can increase confidence and a sense of well-being.[80] A negative environment can have the opposite effect.

It is difficult to assist an older person, especially a family member, with the decision of whether to stay in his or her own environment or to opt for an assisted living arrangement. Of course, if the person has been diagnosed with a progressive illness such as Alzheimer's disease or Parkinson's, it is more cut and dried. As with Aunt Rose, it can be favorable for the person to remain in a familiar environment as long as possible. With certain diseases however, the environment itself becomes threatening and the person does not always recognize where he or she is. Then, it is time for a change for the sake of safety, if nothing else.

As for her mother, the signs were staring Virginia in the face. It was becoming increasingly clear that Alice was unable to care for herself. Virginia only had to face it. In addition to becoming lost, not opening the mail, not eating much of anything, letting food rot in the refrigerator, generally not picking anything up (there was a cleaning service, so this was not obvious) and not seeing anyone for days at a time, these next things tipped the scale.

Alice had always been a fastidious person, especially about hygiene. When Virginia was growing up, she was always dusting the furniture and caring for the house. Virginia's next visit to her mother was unannounced. She knocked at the door in the early afternoon and to her surprise, her mother answered the door, still in her pajamas. While she was taking a shower, Virginia started to make the bed and noticed the sheets were dirty and her nightclothes were soiled. She didn't know what to make of this, so she confronted her with the issue. Alice seemed a bit confused as though she hadn't noticed. Virginia put her things in the laundry, deciding not to take any action for the moment. If there was a problem, she had been good at hiding it up until then.

Another sign Virginia noticed on that occasion was her mother had difficulty getting out of her chair and needed some assistance. Virginia was afraid of hurting her or pulling too hard. When she did get up, she was unsteady and shuffled along. She often said she was afraid of falling and breaking a hip. *When you break a hip, you're done*, she would say. Of course Virginia was worried, too. Those who are not afraid of falling actually reduce the risk.[81] This was not Alice; she knew she would have a fall. This was a scary situation and Virginia didn't know what to do as she had had no experience with people who could not move well. She needed help. It was getting to the stage where Alice would need full-time supervision or care of some sort. She had always been a private person and did not like the thought of having a stranger forced into her space, telling her what to do. Her daughter needed to please her and also be sure she would remain healthy.

At first, Virginia found it difficult to accept that any of her immediate relatives, especially one of her parents, could be in need of full time nursing care. Could it really be that her mother, on whom she had always depended, needed this much help? She felt powerless and didn't know what to do. She had no siblings or any other relatives to consult and she was in denial over the whole situation. It turned out that this attitude was not helpful for either of them in the long run.

Virginia finally decided it was necessary to employ full-time staff to be with her mother. This decision was very unpopular. Virginia considered advertising for live-in help, but she still lived a long distance away and was unsure how she would monitor this person. She has since heard horror stories about caregivers who have extorted possessions, money and even property from their senior charges. She is relieved

now that she did not make that choice. In the end, she used
a staffing agency that had been recommended by some local
friends. Her mother got along with a couple of the caregivers,
but there was no guarantee they would be available. Alice's
reaction to those she didn't like was to insult them or throw
things at them. Sometimes, she would bang the furniture and
hurl the china at her caregiver. She had a valuable collection
of antique furniture of which she was very proud. The fact
that she would damage it in anger was distressing to Virginia.
At the time, she didn't understand her mother's behavior.
Later she began to appreciate that her mother was venting her
fear and frustration at losing control of her life and faculties
to which she was desperately clinging. At the time Virginia
didn't know what to think.

Virginia called frequently and, at least, had the comfort
of knowing someone was always there keeping an eye on her
mother, making sure she was taking her medications, bathing
and eating regularly. Sometimes during their telephone
conversations Alice would appear to be perfectly fine, as
Virginia had always known her. They would talk about the
grandchildren and she would relate some gossip from her
building. Other times, it was as if she was someone else
altogether. Alice wasn't sure where she was or why there was
a stranger in her apartment and she was easily disoriented. She
always recognized Virginia as her daughter but sometimes
would confuse the children with each other. It was becoming
increasingly clear she had problematic medical issues.
Virginia started to wonder how much longer she could stay in
her apartment even with full-time staff and a nurse who visited
twice a week. She knew her mother was unhappy with the
situation, but she didn't know what she could do to make it
better. The issue was compounded in her mind because there
was no one else to give an opinion and she was on her own.

The distance between mother and daughter was
becoming defeating. As it was clearly not an option for
Virginia to move closer to her mother, she decided it would

be best to move her mother closer to her. This was a difficult decision for several reasons. For Virginia, it meant a lot of organizing and traveling across the country - not to mention the expense. For Alice, it meant taking her away from the environment she knew and from the familiar surroundings which are good for confidence in both physical and cognitive arenas, as Virginia had already observed from her aunt.[82] There was no one close to her mother who would check on her and surely she would be less lonely if she were closer to her only child and her family. So, in the end, Virginia decided Alice had to move. She didn't ask her mother if that was what she wanted. She approached it as though she was coming to visit only on a permanent basis. The big question in her mind was where her mother should live. Alice had already made the decision some years earlier to move into an environment where she would receive care. Virginia could only suppose it was reassuring to her mother to know someone – anyone - would be there to take care of her should the need arise. She must have felt she could not rely on her daughter as she was not near by, and perhaps Alice didn't want to be a burden. Who knows?

Virginia grappled with the idea that her mother could have come to live with her and her family in California. Alice had been out to visit once before, accompanied by her nurse. Virginia realized there were a couple of problems with that idea. Her house was not conducive to someone in her mother's situation. It was multi-level and, since by this time Alice was unsteady on her feet and had to be assisted with getting up from a chair, going up and down stairs would be impossible. *Should I have thought of that when I bought the house in the first place?* Virginia wondered. Maybe, but she didn't. Another problem was her mother's supervision. Virginia would not be available to be there all the time and that meant hiring a caregiver. That would be all right but there was no room for someone to live in the house and how would she manage at night? In addition to her other concerns, Alice's medical issues seemed to be increasing. The whole prospect was turning into an ordeal. In the end, a care facility seemed to be the best choice. Virginia would still be able to visit her often and keep a closer eye on her. With two children at home, location and convenience of her accommodation was a factor. She would have to be able to juggle visiting her mother, her children's activities and her own schedule.

Another issue was the time factor. It was as though once she had decided her mother should move, it needed to happen right away. The move was planned and executed in fairly short order and there was not much time to research living accommodations for Alice. She needed to find a place for her to live *now*. At the time, care facilities in the area were not places where Virginia had spent time or had prior reason to research. A friend gave her the name of a care facility that had a good reputation. It was part of a corporate chain and, when she first visited it, her immediate impression was that the facility felt like a hospital, not that she had any idea what to expect since she did not have any point of comparison. There was a nurse's station, with a cluster of people in wheel chairs in front of it and carts with supplies sitting in the hall. Occasionally, a loud speaker would blare out someone's name to call extension 121 or 512. *How intrusive,* she thought. She tried to imagine herself living there and she couldn't. It was quite a different story from the place in Florida. This was a full nursing facility rather than individual apartments or an assisted living facility. There were no locks on the doors and, seemingly, very little privacy. Time was still a big issue and she thought it would be temporary until she had time to really look around. In hindsight, Virginia wished she had taken more time to plan this event.

Virginia somewhat timidly flew to Florida to bring her mother back with her on the plane. It was a little strange to think she actually had the power to do this. They packed up Alice's possessions and arranged for movers to clear out her apartment. Things were going along smoothly until sometime during the flight when Alice suddenly gathered her purse and coat, got up and started off down the aisle of the plane.

Virginia asked her where she was going and she replied she was going home. After some discussion, she was convinced that she could not get off an airplane at thirty thousand feet and so she sat back down. Virginia was frightened by this episode but also thought it a little amusing. As she looked back on it later, she realized that it was another attempt by her mother to stay in control of her life.[83]

In the end, moving her again did not seem to be a good option. Virginia was afraid she would become even more disoriented. Although she felt a little strange having her mother so close but not actually living with her, she rationalized it by telling herself that her mother had chosen to move to a community that offered the same type of care should it be needed. The time problem was mainly due to her own denial of her mother's needs. Had she accepted the situation earlier, she would have had more time to investigate. In the end, she was lucky because the facility she chose worked out just fine. She tried to visit her mother in her new home as often as possible. Her room was pleasant enough. Some accommodations were doubles but Alice had her own room. Virginia had some of her furniture moved in along with some pictures with the hope she would feel more at home. Sometimes, Virginia would find Alice in the activities room making cookies or doing an art project. One year, she made a turkey out of clay at Thanksgiving. In reality, she watched the activities director make the clay turkey but at least she was out of her room and with other people. She was interacting and beginning to feel a sense of belonging or at least that's what Virginia thought. When she would wheel her mother down to the dining room for dinner, Alice would point out her table each time and tell her daughter who would be coming to join her. She had always been a little nosey about other people's business so this proximity gave her the perfect opportunity. The staff encouraged the community aspect and the socialization.

Once Virginia had her mother installed in the care facility, she started to look around at the other residents. Most of them seemed to be there long term. She remembered one lady celebrating her 102nd birthday shortly after Alice arrived. The old lady was pleasant to talk to, although she couldn't hear very well. She was able to propel herself around in her wheelchair at a pretty good clip. She always showed up for happy hour and enjoyed her highball before dinner. Virginia tried to visit at that time because it seemed more social, but she could not help but notice very few other residents had family members who visited. She persisted with her visits, but she found herself thrown into an unfamiliar environment. The facility was full of other old people, to whom she couldn't relate, waiting to die. She began to think the whole place was a little depressing.

What was it like for these people? Virginia didn't wonder at the time. She was so happy to have her mother in a safe place she didn't think to ask how Alice was feeling about the situation. There may also have been an element of relief - she wouldn't have to look after her mother all the time and she was so busy. She didn't have time to care for her mother every minute, and she couldn't just drop everything. She did wonder if Alice felt abandoned in a strange place. Looking back, Virginia could see that the community aspect of the facility and the sense of belonging were of utmost importance. Nevertheless, the staff reported Alice cried a lot and continuously called out her daughter's name; sometimes she refused to get up. The doctor said she had a mild form of dementia and was suffering from depression. He ordered some medication which he thought would help but Virginia's impression was the medication seemed to make her more forgetful and disorientated than ever. Virginia wasn't sure if this was a good idea, but at least Alice seemed a little happier and less anxious.

Although Alice was not in a locked unit, none of the residents left the facility by themselves. Most of the residents

were in wheel chairs; hardly anyone walked. The staff seemed
to prefer it that way. Virginia supposed it was easier to keep
track of them and they were less likely to wander off and get
lost. The few who did walk were stooped over a walker in
an unnatural position. Man is designed to walk erectly, but
gravity plays its part and, with the loss of power and agility
associated with aging, we tend to shrink and become more
stooped as we are pulled closer to the ground. This is a typical
image of an older person. In some cases, the "senile posture"
is a matter of habit and can, with conviction, be corrected.[84]
Plus, inactivity leads to loss of muscle mass which makes
the person appear frail and thin.[85] They become all skin
and bone; not what we think of as healthy and robust. This
appearance contributes to the "cactus" image making these
people less likely to be touched. We hear a lot in the media
about osteoporosis or brittle bones and about medications
which might prevent this condition; they might even reverse
it. Inactivity cannot be good for bones or muscles.[86] After
years in a wheelchair, the opportunity for brittle bones can only
be increased. Does this mean arms and legs should not move
or be moved? Are they safer if they just stay in place? Alice
certainly had no intention of moving around any more than
necessary so she would only get weaker.

Virginia was able to visit her mother on most days.
Usually, the afternoon was the best time because the routine
at the facility was very busy in the morning. Now that she
was seeing Alice more regularly, she began to notice a lot of
things about her mother's aging process that bothered her. She
could see right through her mother's skin. All kinds of veins
had surfaced and her skin looked like a thin membrane. The
skin is the largest organ of the body and her mother's was
disappearing before her eyes. Virginia wondered if it was
going to eventually disappear and one day, everything inside
her arms and legs would fall out! Of course, this wasn't going
to happen. Surely if such things actually happened, one would
hear about it in the press. Could she damage her mother's skin
by touching it? She wondered; so, she didn't touch her.

Sometimes, Alice would complain of a pain and gasp for breath. *Take a deep breath,* her daughter would say, as she had been told when she was a child. The elderly do seem to breathe in a shallow way. Cardiovascular exercise encourages deeper breathing; lying in bed or sitting in a wheelchair all day does not. For the inactive, such as the elderly, shallow breathing becomes the norm.[87]

Virginia also noticed their conversations had become quite limited. Alice's decline in terms of movement – the wheel chair showed up pretty soon – and in terms of memory – the dementia – made it appear that she didn't care about any of the problems Virginia was having with her own family at the time. She would not remember if Virginia had been there the day before. When Virginia tried to explain to her what was going on, or to ask her advice, she had little to say. Virginia quickly found herself growing impatient with what felt like an ever increasing distance between them. Talking to her was impossible and Virginia would become frustrated with her mother when she would not pay attention. Soon she would be nodding off! The tendency to easily fall asleep leads to the appearance of inattention. Actually, most of the residents sitting in their wheelchairs often appeared to fall asleep. At a certain age, although the amount of REM sleep[88] diminishes, the time spent dozing off increases.[89] Virginia had certainly noticed her aunt spending more time sleeping in her later years. Most of the residents were on some kind of regular medication that may also have contributed to drowsiness. Although Virginia knew these things, they were suffocated in her mind by the frustrations she was experiencing with Alice.

A physical result of not walking is increased weakness and this certainly was the appearance of many of the residents. Inactivity can also lead to stiffness and/or pain in the joints which gives the appearance of frailty and lack of ability. This was yet another source of annoyance about Virginia's mother. Alice never did move quickly and used the excuse of having small feet and thin ankles to justify her lack of physical activity. Virginia became impatient with her slowness and inability to participate. It was almost a relief when her mother moved into the wheelchair. Transferring her in or out of the wheelchair was a problem, but at least she could be pushed along at a reasonable pace. Alice was perfectly content to be waited on hand and foot, as she put it. Her general weakness did seem to increase with the wheelchair, though. Soon, she was unable to stand unassisted or bear her own weight on her legs. For Virginia, the vision of her mother's weakness evoked emotions somewhere between sadness, pity and, worst of all, revulsion.

The loss of function bothered Alice more than she let on. She had lost her independence to the extent that she had to rely on someone else for everything. This was a difficult transition, moving from complete independence to none at all. For Alice, the transition was gradual and partly self-imposed in that she had always led a sedentary life style and her tendency to simply sit in a chair increased as she got older. For others, the change can be sudden, brought on by a stroke or another illness. This can cause what appears to be a personality change. An outgoing person can become introverted and unwilling to talk. Alice went from being fastidious to careless. Her prized possessions suddenly didn't matter and she would damage treasured things in frustration and anger. The fear of being alone or left in pain to die can make the older or sick person irritable. It was hard for Virginia to continually have patience with this behavior, even if it was justified and understood.

Sometimes, Virginia and the children would take Alice out for lunch or ice cream. On holidays, they would bring her to the house. She was in the wheelchair by this time and the whole outing proved to be an ordeal to which Virginia did not look forward. It was not that she didn't want to have her mother with the family, but the mechanics of the outing were daunting. She was, of course, concerned her mother might have an accident such as falling out of her wheelchair. What if she had to go to the bathroom? She wore adult diapers that were sent along with her, but Virginia would have to change her. This was such a role reversal for the daughter that she felt like a duck out of water.

There were occasions when Alice would complain she wanted to *get out of this place.* Nevertheless, Virginia found she was taking her mother out less often and, when they did go out somewhere, Alice was anxious to get back. She felt more secure in the facility than she did when she was out with her daughter. That suited Virginia just fine. As the years went on, Alice grew more forgetful and confused. Virginia had become accustomed to having brief conversations and not really being able to talk or ask advice. She wondered how this happened and what it had been like for her mother. Was the care facility another nail in the coffin, so to speak? As she didn't have to do anything for herself, did she deteriorate faster? It was really hard to say if that was the case. At the time, Virginia thought there was little choice.

They had never been a very touchy-feely family, so a peck on the cheek was as close as Virginia came to touching he mother. As there was nothing to talk about, the visits seemed like a burden so Virginia felt less and less inclined to visit and, when she did, she found it hard to keep her temper.[90] Her frustration grew until she became angry with her mother for being the way she was. Virginia couldn't understand why it seemed like she had lost someone in her life and yet, she was still there. Left with no way to fix the situation, she wondered if other people felt like that. The other visitors at her mother's facility seemed to behave in a civil manner but there were very few other visitors. In fact, she could remember only one regular person. Why was that? Were their families miles away? Did they not have families? Did the families not care? Did they find it distressing, as she did, to see their loved ones incapacitated? She asked herself these questions later, but at the time, although she thought it strange, she brushed it off.

After a couple of months of Alice being in the care facility, Virginia was contacted by the facility manager who suggested they take advantage of the services of a massage therapist who visited the facility regularly. Her mother, to her knowledge, had never had a massage in her life. She didn't really like to be touched because she always thought she might catch something. Why would she want to start now? Still, Virginia thought the extra personal attention might be good for her. So, she agreed. There was no point in asking her mother if she wanted a massage because she would have said *no*. At first, Alice didn't understand why this strange woman was visiting her or what she wanted. The therapist was unobtrusive and worked her way up to touching her gradually. After a few months, Virginia was getting reports that her mother was enjoying the light touch and the attention. So, this was a success despite her upbringing without touch.

Looking back, Virginia realized she was not very compassionate toward her mother. She did not fully understand what Alice was going through nor did she want to. It has taken Virginia years to come to an appreciation, which is still far from complete, of the situation faced by all of us toward the end of life as we know it. The real questions are: What can be done to make this situation more tolerable? How can the quality of life be improved? How do we go about improving it? Inadvertently, answering these questions became a quest. Like her mother, the idea of a massage had never crossed Virginia's mind. In fact, she thought of massage as a little repulsive - a stranger touching her. She had no idea what a massage would be like. She had no desire to find out. She didn't want to touch other people and she didn't want them to touch her. Years later she would find herself in exactly the reverse position.

Chapter 5

Learning to Touch

Although Virginia Goodrich's upbringing was not exactly the huggy type, that doesn't mean it was cold. She always knew her parents loved her and wished for nothing less than her happiness. They were sorry she lived so far away for so many years but, if she was happy, they did not try to influence her to move closer. The lack of physical touch in the family is something Virginia believes that she inadvertently passed on to her children but, when they were young, she didn't know the difference. That changed in a dramatic manner when her daughter became ill.

After Virginia's father died she returned home with her husband and their two beautiful, bright and happy young daughters. A few months after the funeral she was standing in the kitchen of their west London home one morning when she received a call from her daughter's school. A calm English voice announced that her twelve year old, Nicola, had collapsed during gym class. She rushed to the school to find they had called an ambulance because they had been unable to revive her. *What on earth could be the matter?* she wondered. *Maybe it was something she ate,* she rationalized as she navigated Hammersmith roundabout toward the hospital. She wasn't really worried.

Her husband joined her at the hospital and they found Nicola in casualty. Little could they imagine what had actually happened. Nicola had suffered a type of stroke and was unconscious. Virginia was kind of numb all over. She couldn't even think straight enough to ask questions. Somewhere deep inside she knew her daughter would be all right. She held Nicola's hand and kissed her on the cheek. Nicola tried to kiss back. That was encouraging. Virginia knew they were communicating, sensing Nicola knew her mother was there.

Nicola was transferred from casualty to an intensive care ward. A blood vessel in her head had burst and she remained in a coma. The doctors didn't seem to know much or do much. Virginia and her husband were told to wait so they sat by her bedside. Virginia was in uncontrollable tears most of the time; she could not believe it was her beautiful daughter lying there.

In her somewhat sheltered childhood, Virginia had not experienced people being hospitalized or doctors and medical staff, other than of course childbirth and her younger daughter's overnight stay to have her tonsils removed. Her father's illness had been her most extended hospital exposure but she had been in the shadow of her mother who took on the doctor interface position. Her high school job as a hospital volunteer was to take water pitchers around to the rooms. As she had no real contact with the patients and certainly did not talk to any doctors, in her mind, this was not a real hospital experience. She felt like a fish out of water. She was in the way when the nurse came to check Nicola's vital signs. All she could do was sit in the corner. She couldn't go home. What if Nicola woke up? A friend was caring for Nicola's younger sister, Charlotte, so she stayed by Nicola's bed as much as possible.

The days and nights dragged on and nothing much changed. Virginia was still confident her daughter would be all right. In the late afternoon she drove home through the busy London traffic to spend some time with Charlotte. It was nearly dark by then and peering through her tears and the light drizzle she could barely see the reflections of the passing lights in the wet streets. To complicate matters, Charlotte had a friend staying at their house because her parents had gone away on vacation. Virginia didn't think it was fair to subject the friend to hospital visits so both girls stayed away. It was hard on Charlotte.

Finally, one afternoon, Nicola opened her eyes. She was very sleepy and didn't want to talk, but she was awake! Virginia was thankful for that. She kissed her and hugged her and held her hand. Nicola complained of a headache that wouldn't go away. Virginia told the doctors but again they didn't say much. Nicola was moved into a ward and Virginia was instantly aware of how noisy it was. She was terrified her daughter would have a repeat stroke with the excessive noise contributing to it. Again, the doctors were unconcerned.

A few days later, they discovered Nicola was paralyzed on her left side. Virginia was horrified. The doctors were non-committal about the paralysis. They said the blood clot in her head would dissolve and she would regain her function. They suggested she could have physiotherapy after she left the hospital but it wasn't really necessary. Virginia felt the doctors were not being pro-active enough but she didn't know where to turn.

After Nicola had been in the hospital for about six weeks, they were told she was ready to go home. For Virginia, this was both good and bad. She had no experience with someone with a brain injury and, except for walking, she expected her daughter to return to normal right away. She would do her schoolwork and watch her favorite TV shows and play with her sister. Virginia couldn't have been more wrong. When Nicola did come home, there was the problem of the stairs. Virginia encouraged her to climb the stairs without being carried, as she had practiced at the hospital. Virginia followed behind holding her hand and, as she was only twelve, could have prevented her from falling. What would they have done if she had been an adult? Virginia was to find out later.

All Nicola wanted to do was to sit on the sofa. Virginia encouraged her to watch TV, but she wasn't interested and she certainly wasn't ready to go back to school. At first Virginia read to her – classics mostly like *The Secret Garden*. Later she was able to copy work from her classmates but concentrating exhausted her. What Virginia did not appreciate was the time required for a brain injury to heal. Although it seemed that Nicola was sitting around doing nothing, she was actually very busy. Internally, she was processing, reconnecting and healing. This took time. Virginia put most of the other things in her life on hold and waited. Nicola's friends came to visit, which was a good stimulus for her. Their visits made her feel wanted and missed and it felt less like she had dropped off the face of the earth.

Virginia remained confident Nicola would regain her strength and mental abilities and return to school. The school's headmistress came to visit and assured them Nicola should take her time and return when she was ready so they stayed home and continued to wait. A few years earlier, a friend invited Virginia to volunteer for a Riding for the Disabled program designed for children who had cerebral palsy. The children would come from their school and ride on giant horses led around the indoor ring by the volunteers. It took three volunteers for each horse. Something about the rhythm of the horse's gait relaxed the muscles of the children. They loved it. Virginia got to know some of the children during the few years that she worked in the program. She had not had any contact with the disabled prior to that experience and, reflecting on plight of those children, perhaps it was God's way of preparing her for having her own disabled child. It did help her emotionally. She could relate Nicola's condition to those children and somehow it became more bearable.

Nicola got better slowly, but it was so slow that it was almost imperceptible. Then, one day, Virginia realized she was nearly back to normal and it might be time for her to return to school. The school made a lot of concessions and she managed to complete all her classes. Her friends were all glad to see her back. Virginia heaved a sigh of relief, glad to have that chapter closed, or so she thought.

Little did Virginia realize the nightmare of her child's health problem was in its infancy. The doctor's reported that, although Nicola had recovered from the stroke, the cause of the stroke was still in her brain and the whole incident would very likely recur. The culprit was a collection of malformed blood vessels, very thin and spidery – a birth defect - which had ruptured due to the high pressure of the blood traveling through the brain. The medical name was arterioveinous malformation (AVM). Often, these things can be surgically removed, but in her case it was too risky because of the location of the AVM, deep in her brain. The major immediate concern was a repeat bleed. The doctors did not have a specific cause for the bleed. It could happen if she was lying in bed or riding her bike. There were no restrictions on her activities. Life should go on as normal.

Normal! How can things be normal when there is a volcano in my daughter's head waiting to erupt and send red rivers flowing into her brain? Something had to be done! The doctors suggested a relatively new procedure, the Gamma Knife, which had been used to treat peripheral tumors in the brain but never on something as deep as Nicola's AVM. It had also not been used on a child. The family agreed, as it seemed like the only available option at the time, and they nervously traveled by train north to Sheffield to a hospital where the procedure would be performed. Nicola appeared cheerful and had her photograph taken in front of the bulbous white machine that resembled a mini-reactor. The procedure seemed to last forever and when Nicola emerged the doctors said it would take some time to tell if it had been successful or not. So, they waited again.

The doctors continued to maintain the AVM could not be removed safely using surgery and refused to take any action. At this stage Nicola's quality of life was not good due to constant severe headaches. This was about the time Virginia started looking for second opinions, and third and fourth. The search led her far and wide, from Europe to South America to the United States. A move back to the U.S. fitted into their agenda for a number of reasons. They had always planned on the girls finishing their schooling there. Some friends had recently moved from London to California and Virginia had some cousins in the same area. A neurosurgeon near San Francisco was specializing in treating conditions such as Nicola's and, with the help of a physician friend and a referral from the surgeon in London, they contacted him. The new doctor felt there was no choice but to remove the offending cluster of blood vessels in Nicola's head. The blood was leaking into her brain, causing the pain which sent them to the emergency room on more than one occasion, and it was only a matter of time before the AVM erupted again with unknown results.

Virginia felt relieved and thankful someone had finally agreed to take action. It was five years after the initial bleed before the surgery was performed. During those years, the family tried to go on as normal, but there was always the ever-present cloud of disaster looming. The routine had come to include trips to doctors' offices and emergency rooms and a lot more waiting.

When the day of the surgery finally came, everyone was nervous as this was a big step with an uncertain outcome. Virginia didn't have any emotion, just numbness and an impatience to get it over with. She felt helpless sitting in the hospital waiting room during the long operation. Just waiting again! Her whole body had shut down so she wasn't aware of the people around her, the time passing or eating. It seemed odd that she was so alone, without any support around her. Nicola's father and her sister were both in England and her cousins could not come to the hospital. Her mother was of course no help at all. So there she was, waiting. She felt very responsible, much more so than when her father was dying. Somehow, her mother had been the responsible party then, not her. This time was different; it was her child. At the same time, she was aware the outcome was in the hands of the doctors and there was nothing she could do.

Virginia got little information during the six-hour surgery. A psychiatrist who had been following Nicola stopped by to visit with her and someone may have come out to give her an update, but it all became a bit hazy. Virginia's major concern was, of course, that her daughter would survive the surgery. She didn't doubt for a moment she would. She had full confidence in skill of the surgeon as she did in Nicola's determination not to die. The other concern was whether it would be successful or not. Would the doctors be able to remove the blood vessels causing the problem? Virginia did not think past that point. It was as though she was revisiting the wait in Sheffield but that procedure had not been life threatening as was the surgery. The drama had heightened as the stakes increased. She didn't think about what she was feeling or about what she was supposed to be feeling. She knew they would get through this.

Nicola did come through the operation and Virginia next saw her in the intensive care unit. The operation had been successful and she was out of danger. Relief! She was there for a few days. What Virginia didn't know, until she was moved to a ward, was her daughter was again paralyzed on the left side. Virginia was still so elated over the results of the surgery that she could not take on any other aspects. Gradually, it dawned on her they would have to deal with the paralysis again. She felt sad seeing Nicola in a wheelchair and trying to walk and wondered what the doctors would say this time. Would her function mysteriously come back on its own like it had the last time? They were not as optimistic as before. Different doctors, different approach, she reasoned. Nicola started physical and occupational therapy at the hospital; progress was slow.

Virginia was certain Nicola would return to normal and be able to return to school as before but the doctors were non-committal as were the therapists. All they would say was each person was different and much depended on how hard she was prepared to work. She was fitted with a cumbersome brace for her left leg (ankle-foot orthotic – AFO). It was intended to keep her ankle bent at a right angle. She also had a brace for her left arm and hand that was to be worn at night. It was supposed to keep her fingers from curling. Virginia realized her daughter's recovery was going to be more of a battle than she had imagined, but she was resolved they would succeed.

Nicola remained in the hospital for about two months following the surgery. Now that Virginia felt that her daughter's health was under control and she wasn't in immanent danger of dying, her attention turned to coping with the home-coming from the hospital. Virginia realized leaving Nicola alone could be a problem and she would need assistance with most daily tasks they take for granted. As the discharge date approached, sometime in the late spring, Virginia became increasingly anxious. Nicola was now seventeen and much more of an adult size than when she was twelve so physically supporting her was more difficult. Other than the riding with the disabled program, Virginia had no experience with helping people who were unable to function. The hospital was more interested in making sure she understood how and when Nicola should wear her braces than in instruction on the day-to-day problems that might occur in helping her to move around. Virginia also wondered if her own emotional involvement would hinder her abilities and judgment around Nicola's activities. It would be hard to remain objective.

The more she thought about all the potential problems, the more worried Virginia became. She wasn't sure exactly how her anxiety manifested itself. A few weeks before the discharge date, she decided to go on a retreat for a few days to a Buddhist center, Green Gulch Farm, located north of San

Francisco. There was a fairly set routine of mundane tasks with a little time off during the day. Quiet and reflection were intended. She found some of the tasks frustrating and she cried a lot. Finally, she realized this was exactly what she needed and, despite the frustrations, she left refreshed and ready to face whatever was to come.

Once they got home from the hospital and settled into a routine, life was not as difficult as Virginia had imagined and she heaved a sign of relief. She continued to be saddened at seeing her daughter this way, but she also remained confident Nicola's situation was only temporary and her function would return to at least near normal as it had before. The continuing rounds of doctors' visits, combined with physical, occupational and speech therapists, served to heighten their optimism or at least that was how they began. The first round of therapy was at a local hospital which they attended twice a week. Finally, when the insurance company decided enough was enough, Nicola was transferred to a state-run program for children under the age of twenty-two. This program provided therapy in a different location but under the supervision of the same doctor; progress was slow. There were exercises to be done at home, which Nicola did religiously, and she continued to wear her ankle and hand braces. They would often meet other children who had encountered some difficulty and Virginia noticed she did not have an aversion to talking to them, as she would have had a few years prior. Her attitude toward the disabled had changed, seemingly as a result of her personal involvement with her daughter's condition and treatment.

By the fall, Nicola was able to return to school on a limited schedule. She was walking unassisted, except for her ankle brace and a cane. She took her time getting from one class to another and the school and her classmates were all very tolerant. Her exceptional sense of humor helped to ease the discomfort of those around her. The schedule allowed for the therapy visits, so they continued well into the winter with the same set of therapists. One day, the physical therapist announced she was no longer seeing any change in Nicola's walking and this was probably as good as it was going to get. The therapist didn't feel she could justify continuing the therapy and essentially, they were sent packing. Nicola was very upset and insisted on leaving immediately. Virginia was crestfallen. She could not accept what the therapist was telling them; it was still early days, she reasoned. Sometimes, she felt as though there was a switch in her daughter's brain and if only they could find it, they could turn everything back on. She held onto that thought for several years.

It was time for another retreat to recover from this discouraging news. While Virginia had been at Green Gulch Farm, she had heard about another rejuvenating place called the Esalen Institute.[91] She had been told they offered classes in a variety of self-help and healing modalities which sounded like just what she needed so she called and asked for a catalog. When it arrived, Virginia eagerly poured through it finding a long list of workshops describing people and techniques, none of which she recognized. What were things like Gestalt Practice[92] and Hanna Somantics?[93] Some of them sounded more than a little scary and she was nervous she might be signing up for more self-discovery than she really wanted. She had to do something however and, since she was feeling so disappointed with the medical community for sending them home, she decided she was game for anything.

Esalen was indeed a beautiful place, located in Big Sur, California, overlooking the Pacific. Founded by two idealistic young men in the 1960s, the area was once inhabited by the Esalen Indian tribe, thus the name. The grounds were extensive and included simple accommodations, a lodge with a dining room, which served healthy buffet style meals three times a day, numerous rooms where workshops were conducted as well as an art studio and a meditation building. There were hot springs on the property with very hot water that came right out of the rock along the cliff. You could relax in the large outside baths in the fog or under the stars. The three-day class Virginia signed up for was entitled "Qui Gong." She had no idea what that meant or what she was going to do. It was beautiful weather so the class was held outside on a lawn and everyone, except Virginia, was dressed in loose, flowing clothing and many wore flat sandals. They made her tight little shoes look uncomfortable. The class started out a little oddly involving a lot of balancing, slow movements and waving of arms. Perhaps it was their calm assurance and acceptance that drew her in and, by the end of the three days, much to her surprise, she felt energized and positive again.

It was at Esalen that Virginia first heard about the Feldenkrais Method.[94] She was in the family-style dining room, telling her problems to a woman she had never met before, when the stranger suddenly blurted out, "Feldenkrais Method, you should try the Feldenkrais Method." Virginia pondered all the 'w' words – *what is it, who does it, where do I find it???* A woman named Harriet Goslins was a practitioner of the work and, from time to time, she held workshops at Esalen. Virginia decided they couldn't wait for the next time so, after some maneuvering, she obtained Harriet's phone number and called. Harriet patiently listened to Virginia's story and was very sympathetic, especially with her frustration with the therapy which had just been terminated. Virginia later discovered other people experience similar frustrations with the system. She felt better after talking on the phone to Harriet who agreed to see Nicola if they could come to Laguna Beach, California, where she lived. Luckily, they were close enough to drive and were able to stay in a fairly inexpensive local hotel.

Harriet appeared to be a warm, friendly person with the same kind of air as those Virginia had met at Esalen. The first thing she did was to discard the brace on Nicola's ankle, reasoning that if the function of her leg was going to change, it needed freedom to find its own way, or at least that was the impression she gave. Most of the work was done behind closed doors while Virginia waited in another room or went back to the hotel. It was all very mysterious. Harriet worked with Nicola for two days and at the end of each session they appeared to display the changes. The first thing to change was Nicola's smile which had drooped on the left side. It was now nearly equal and her left eye was also much more open than before. These were permanent changes according to Harriet. The basis of the Feldenkrais Method was to use movements to rewire the brain so the body could move in the way it was designed to function. It meant re-learning some very basic things. Virginia was naturally skeptical, but at the end of the short time, Nicola did stand more erect and was much more confident. Nicola had also stopped using her ankle and hand braces and was moving more naturally. The most encouraging thing of all was to have someone tell them there was room for change so they went home feeling uplifted asking when they could come again.

As Nicola continued working with Harriet, Virginia began to be drawn into the mysteries of this therapy. She couldn't help being curious about what was going on and how they were achieving results. Results in this case were changes in her daughter's physical function. She decided if she was going to be of any help to Nicola she had to understand her therapy and that meant experiencing it herself. Mother and daughter soon found themselves back in Laguna Beach to attend a week-long session in Harriet's own version of the Feldenkrais Method, now called Cortical Field Reeducation® (CFR). Virginia should come along as moral support for Nicola, or so said Harriet. Yes, she agreed, moral support was good but she was also beginning to be fascinated by this newfound level of human involvement, the like of which she had not before experienced.

The first workshop with Harriet included a dozen or so people in the living room of a bright house overlooking the Pacific. The room had been cleared of furniture so everyone could find a place on the floor. In fact the workshop seemed to consist mainly of a lot of lying on the floor with closed eyes and making small, isolated movements with one or another part of the body. With the soothing sound of the waves against the rocks below, the group followed Harriet's directions on how to make each movement. One expression that came up frequently was *hands on*. At first, Virginia wasn't sure what that meant. *Can you put hands on?* Harriet would ask one of her assistants, or, *Would you like me to put hands on?* someone would ask her. *No, thank you*, she invariably said, when she realized this expression meant physically touching her. She didn't know these people, she didn't really want them touching her and she didn't want to be pushed or squeezed. She might catch something! Of course, that was her mother, Alice, talking.

The other people in the workshop all also seemed to have some grave problem from which they were recovering. Virginia considered herself somewhat special, as she had not personally had any physical problems and had only joined as an extension of Nicola to give her support. She was eager to observe and learn but not too sure about the participation part. Little did she realize the extent to which she would soon become involved.

The workshop started with everyone sitting in a circle on the floor. Virginia was unaccustomed to this posture and soon became stiff and uncomfortable. She moved to a chair. No one seemed to notice. Moving around the circle each person introduced him or herself and stated why they were there and what they hoped to accomplish at the workshop. Virginia said she was accompanying her daughter. That was not good enough. Why was *she* there and what was *she* hoping to get out of it? This made her pause to think. She was hoping, of course, to see her daughter improve in function and... *hmmmm*; she couldn't come up with anything about herself at that moment. Thankfully, the spotlight moved on to the next person. Throughout the week, the circle had a habit of being repeated and the same question kept coming up. Virginia never did arrive at a meaning for herself during that first week of CFR.® However, she did go home in a different frame of mind. The therapy certainly seemed to be helping

Nicola and Virginia could see her daughter continue to gain confidence. Harriet recalled that, "Over the next year of work, [Nicola] improved her balance and stability and the use of her left leg. She was also able to feel temperature differences on her left arm for the first time."[95]

During the continuing lessons with Harriet – one week was not the end by a long shot – people were continually talking about changing the way the brain communicates with the rest of the body. This was something Virginia had never really thought about too much. She had always taken this delicate communication system pretty much for granted but, suddenly faced with her daughter's malfunctioning system, she started to observe other people's small unnatural movements and postures, which, according to her new instructors, lead to disability later in life. Correcting them was a matter of paying close attention to small movements as directed by the teacher. Once corrected, the body could return to the pain-free and easy-moving state for which it was designed. That sounded good. Considerably more time was spent lying on the floor with closed eyes. Virginia couldn't help peeking to see what Nicola was doing and if she could manage the movements. Sometimes an assistant would help her with a movement but most of the time she was left to find her own way. Virginia tried hard to resist the temptation to watch. It was painful.

During the classes and especially during breaks, which were never often or long enough, Harriet would talk about other therapies which Virginia assumed were her favorites. One was CranioSacral Therapy. This one was intriguing because it focused on the nervous system and it was becoming clear to Virginia that therein lay the answer to her daughter's rehabilitation. She decided to research this therapy and, with Harriet's recommendation, got in touch with the Upledger Institute[96] located in West Palm Beach, Florida. Founded by Dr. John Upledger, the Institute not only offers therapy at its Florida facility but also conducts a range of classes across the USA and abroad. Excited at the thought of learning another approach, she enrolled as a non-professional in an introductory class in her location.

On a Thursday morning in July, Virginia arrived well before 8AM at the hotel in downtown San Francisco. Dodging the suited business types who bustled across the otherwise vacant lobby, she passed the coffee shop which was starting to fill up with breakfast seekers. In the wide hallway outside a suite of conference rooms it was so early the registration table had yet to be set up. When the table was ready, she approached to find nametags neatly arranged in plastic sleeves. The well-groomed young lady asked which class she was taking. "CranioSacral Therapy I" was the title of the class. It was then that she discovered there were five classes all going on at the same time. Along with her nametag, she was given a bulky, spiral bound workbook and instructed to go to a ballroom toward the end of the hall. Virginia was the first one in the ballroom which had been partitioned off to allow for another class in the other half. Twenty or so eight foot tables were set up with chairs along one side. On top of each table was what appeared to be a bright blue air mat, the kind usually found as part of swimming pool flotilla. A table at the back looked the most inviting so she sat down to look through the workbook. It was filled with line-drawing diagrams of body parts: heads, hands, feet and spines with arrows pointing in different directions. She thought it best to start at the beginning in the hope finding a clue to the contents of the forthcoming class. She had brought with her a hard bound book that had arrived at her house a few weeks earlier. Virginia had read through some of it but, like the workbook, it contained physiological terms and diagrams. Although she had done well in basic biology, chemistry and physics in high school, she had assiduously avoided science since then. The terminology was a bit hazy.

People started filtering into the room and soon it was filled with nearly fifty people. A tall woman with long blond hair, tied at the neck, took up a position at the front of the room. She had a little trouble adjusting the volume on the clip-on microphone but after a few squeals she got it. She was to be teaching the class for the next four days and she also introduced approximately ten assistants who would be giving the students individual attention. Starting at the front of the workbook the instructor gradually went through each section in which Virginia scribbled copious notes and added her own drawings. At the end a technique, the teacher did a demonstation and then the group at each table practiced on each other. The blue mats by the tables were placed on top of the tables to lie on when it was each person's turn to be the client. Virginia felt nervous and out of place but, nevertheless, she jumped right in and mastered the concept of the "semi-hydraulic CranioSacral system."[97]   After all, she was motivated.

At the lunch break Virginia wandered out into the lobby to find a large group of tables covered with books, tapes, posters, devices and even a brightly colored skull. People were crowded around and grabbing things as if they were in a feeding frenzy. All the books looked interesting and she recognized a couple of titles from discussions with Harriet. The day ended about 5PM and she drove home, tired, and prepared to return at the same time the next day. On Friday and Saturday the class continued to work through the workbook and, by around 2 o'clock Sunday afternoon, they had covered the whole book. The class ended early on Sunday so people who had come from other parts of the country could catch planes home. The books in the lobby had disappeared by now, but one table remained where they were taking reservations for more classes. As there was a financial incentive to sign up on the spot, Virginia put her name and credit card down for "CranioSacral Therapy II."

The class had been long and exhausting, but very informative with well organized written materials which served as useful memory aids afterward. Virginia had also come away from the class with a protocol which she could immediately put to use. She realized after talking to a few other attendees that nearly everyone else in the room was certified with something to do with health care. There were doctors, dentists, physical therapists, massage therapists and probably other professionals she didn't recognize. By the end, she had made liaisons with other beginners in this therapy and they started a study group to solidify what they had learned. The study group meetings revealed that each person had picked up slightly different things from the same class. They met several times before it became inconvenient but the sessions proved to be invaluable and Virginia was sure this was the therapy that would help her daughter. She had to learn more.

In order to go forward with the CranioSacral training Virginia decided she would have to have some sort of professional standing. Massage therapy seemed to be the best route. A local massage school, The National Holistic Institute[98] in Emeryville, California, had a program that seemed to fit her needs, so she enrolled. The program was 750 hours in duration. *Was that long?* It sounded long. She didn't know. She would be certified in more than one type of massage and also be exposed to numerous other types previously unknown to her. It sounded great. Just what she needed!

The first day reminded her of Harriet. Twenty-three people of all varieties sat around in a circle on the floor and explained why they were there. Virginia tried to remember what she had said but it had faded from her memory. Others were there because they wanted to help people or they were tired of corporate life and wanted to be their own boss or they had been fired and needed a new career and had seen an ad on TV. The course took six months to complete. There was a lot of information on physiology, pathologies, techniques, contra-indications and a host of different modalities.

The first massage class came along so soon. The teacher gave a demonstration and then each student was to find a partner. *Who will partner with me?* Virginia glanced around nervously. A nice looking young girl smiled and they were set. Thank goodness she would not be the last one left!

The next disturbing event was undressing for the massage. At Harriet's classes no one had to take off their clothes. Virginia was very uncomfortable at the thought. She took a deep breath and took off all her clothes behind a sheet that was held up for privacy. She managed to wind the sheet around her body and struggled to get on the massage table, lying there on her back - very stiff and quivering in anticipation of what was to come next. It turned out not to be bad at all and as the classes progressed, she looked forward both to her turn on the table and to giving massages to the other students. Toward the end of the course the students had to interact with the public. This took two forms: a clinic in the massage school which was open to the public and an externship during which they were to give massages in a community setting, pre-arranged either by themselves or the school. Virginia was again very nervous at the thought of her first encounter with a person outside the class. *Would they be judging her?* Of course they would, she was a student. As she gained experience, she also gained confidence bolstered by continually receiving feedback from clients that she had a good touch. She found connecting with perfect strangers in a way previously unfamiliar was as though she could see into their lives and feel all the experiences held in their bodies. At first, the connection was disturbing, but gradually, Virginia realized she could be of service to these strangers and maybe even help them. NHI was very well organized and the course included classes in business as well as learning about the different applications of touch. By the end of the course, she felt confident she could embark on a new profession if she so wished.

During the massage course, Virginia continued to take classes in CranioSacral Therapy and in Cortical Field Re-education.® Other modalities surfaced such as Integrated Awareness,®[99] founded by Lansing Barrett Gresham, and Pranic Healing,[100] a therapy originated in the Philippines and brought to the United States by Choa Kok Sui. By that time Nicola was in college at the University of California Santa Cruz but she took time to travel with Virginia to San Diego for a class in Pranic Healing. That was when they first learned how to see energy. Virginia could actually see the disturbance caused by the electro-magnetic energy field surrounding all living things. She was stunned by this gradual awakening to the condition of others and she wasn't sure what to do with this new-found awareness. She continued to try to help her daughter with her recovery and she would like to think she made a difference. Virginia did begin to feel less isolated than she had been and more connected to people in general although she was still uncertain about how she felt or how this new connection would affect her life. She was about to find out.

A component of the massage school course was to find an externship placement in the community to give the student experience giving regular massages. Recalling her mother having massage when she lived in the care facility and, as she already knew the staff there, Virginia decided to ask the manager if she could give massages to the staff or residents. At first, they weren't sure and said family permission would be necessary if she wanted to work with the residents, but she could come in and give a presentation to the staff about the benefits of massage. She went to the staff dining room armed with all kinds of reasons why it would be good for them to receive massage on a regular basis. Care giving, especially for the elderly, is a high stress job. The residents often complain because they do not feel well and it can be hard working with the dementia patients. Then, there is all the lifting involved with moving patients around. Virginia was confident everyone would be jump at the chance and her calendar would be full. Well, they weren't quite as enthusiastic as she had hoped, but a few did sign up. She brought in her exceedingly heavy new massage table and set up in an empty room. Everything was perfect, exactly as she had been taught at the massage school, as she waited for her first client to arrive. Rosa was a little late and said she only had a few minutes. Virginia did a brief intake with her and asked her to lie down on the table. She was tense, especially her shoulders; Virginia could feel that right away. She complained of pain in her neck and Virginia tried some techniques to relieve it. After about twenty minutes, Rosa said she had to go, but it had helped and she felt better. Virginia was elated; she had actually made a difference. The next client didn't show up at all. Virginia's feeling of joy was diminished, but the third person, an administrator, arrived and was pleased to take a half hour for a massage. She relaxed into it and reaped the benefits of the touch. At the end of the afternoon, Virginia had seen four people and all of them seemed to be grateful and happy.

Continuing to bring her table back and forth for one afternoon each week, Virginia found more often than not, her new clients forgot or their shift had been changed or they just didn't have time. As she walked up and down the hallway, passing the residents in their wheelchairs, she realized they were the ones with whom she wanted to work. Although the staff would certainly benefit, their schedules were problematic and she could see it was the residents who really needed to be touched. With the help of her school, she devised a simple consent form for the resident's family member or conservator to sign and presented it to the facility manager. As she was still a student, there would be no charge so he agreed to send it to the families of those who the staff felt were in the most need. Within a few weeks, she had nine new clients among the residents.

Chapter 6

Who Are You, Who Am I?

When Virginia started working with the residents in the care facility, her first clients were in the Alzheimer's and dementia care wing. Gradually, she began to acquire clients in the other unit. Those in the second group suffered from various ailments and were unable to care for themselves but did not have severe dementia. As these people are all residents of the care facility, they had constant contact with nursing and support staff. At the beginning Virginia wondered what she had to offer them that the staff did not but, over a period of time, she realized the staff worked on their own agenda and had specified tasks related to the care of the residents. The actual wishes of each resident were often over-ridden by the need to get the job done.

What has recently been termed "person-centered care," which caters to the preferences of the recipient, can be difficult to implement in a nursing home setting. The job is necessary, but difficult, and the work environment can be stressful. It seems staff members are often under-trained and generally dissatisfied.[101] Most states require certification to work as an aide (CNA) in a nursing home. However, different states have different certification training and continuing education unit (CEU) requirements.[102] Sometimes a CEU training is offered by the facility, sometimes not. Staff turnover is high and thus, there is little continuity of caregivers. Virginia remembered her mother's stay in the nursing home when her favorite CNA suddenly left for another job which offered better benefits. By necessity, the personal attention administered to the patient is functional, but not holistic; it does not address the whole being or self. Although some of the staff try very hard, there is usually little time for the personal attention we think should occur.[103] Some facilities offer physical and occupational therapy under the same roof. These therapists provide a valuable service in aiding the residents to regain mobility, independence and self-confidence. Still, they also are not trained in a holistic approach. Virginia soon found her new clients responded to her touch, some in ways they had not shown before, but she had to overcome some logistical hurdles.

Virginia realized immediately there was no way she would be able to get any of her new clients onto a massage table. Even if she did, they might fall off and be injured. With a shudder she recalled her father's story of falling off a chiropractor's table. She also discovered that a very short interval of touch would be all any of them could tolerate. Fifteen-minute increments seemed to be about right. She also had to work around the routine in the facility. At first, she came in the morning, but there was a lot of activity at that time of day with bathing, dressing or hair cuts and she soon found her clients could be difficult to track down. She switched to afternoons after lunch and that worked much better.

When Virginia started working with this population, she had had many hours of massage training aimed at working with able-bodied, basically healthy people who may have had an injury or a stiff neck. She had also had hours of training in energy therapy, working with chi, chakras, prana, movement therapy and other healing modalities. Furthermore, she was used to working with a client on some sort of massage table in a quiet atmosphere. Her clients had been able to verbally communicate and give her feedback. No one had ever mentioned how to treat a frail person whose muscle mass had all but disappeared and who would not understand or respond to a request to lie on a table.

Although there are many conditions that cause dementia, Alzheimer's disease (AD) is the most common.[104] The dementia clients varied in degree of involvement. Some were mobile, usually with a walker, and were able to respond verbally and carry on a conversation of sorts. Others were in wheel chairs but were awake and able to use their hands and could also respond verbally, although not necessarily intelligibly. In the latter stages, they were non-responsive, had minimal control of their limbs and, even if sitting in a wheel chair, usually appeared to be asleep.

Amy, perhaps Virginia's most challenging client, walked continually up and down the corridors, in and out of rooms and would not sit for more than a minute. She also talked constantly but, due partially to lack of teeth, she was very difficult to understand. Her actual diagnosis was complex. She suffered from schizophrenia and alternated between kissing and striking out. Her emotions ran the gamut. During the years Virginia worked with her, she would follow her around the building holding her hand, releasing some of her angry energy or calming her aura when she didn't want to be touched. After a fall, Amy was confined to a chair, which was frustrating for her and may have contributed to her decline. She passed away a few years ago. Virginia sometimes wondered what she was actually doing for Amy, but she heard from her conservators that the nurses were grateful for her work because Amy was calmer and easier to handle after her sessions.

Other than this one very mobile lady, Virginia's clients have been stationary. So much so, that she had to devise ways of working with them as she found them, sometimes in bed, sometimes in a wheelchair. This was challenging in terms of her own body mechanics. The beds and wheelchairs were both lower than the massage tables she was accustomed to using and that situation forced her to try a variety of positions including sitting on the floor. Carrying furniture around with her was not practical and chairs were often nowhere to be found. She finally found by kneeling on one knee she could save her back and she could change from one knee to the other when she got tired.

The other challenge Virginia found was all of her clients were frail, wore diapers or had a variety of bags trailing after them, tended to drool quite a bit, could not sit up and would exhibit unexpected jerky movements. She wondered what she could do to help them. She was no longer in school at this stage, but she had mentors to ask and ask she did. The responses varied from: *I've never worked with that* population, to: *I don't know how you can do it. I couldn't work with them.* All this was a little unsettling, but Virginia resolved to carry on. As she continued seeing the same people week in and week out, they seemed to have more faith in her than she did. Even if they could not speak, Virginia could feel their bodies responding to her touch. She found that trying to *massage* their frail bodies was not necessarily a good approach but gently laying her hands in places to which they were drawn by the person's energy worked just fine. She had learned about a light touch and following the body's signals from her training in CranioSacral therapy and this training proved to be invaluable in these circumstances.

Working with clients suffering from Alzheimer's disease was a challenge for Virginia. She had heard the disease described on a radio program as a "gluing up" of the brain. Alzheimer's disease takes its name from Dr. Alois Alzheimer, a German neuropathologist, who lived at the turn of the twentieth century. In 1901, upon examining a fifty-one year old female patient with dementia symptoms which, at the time, were associated with extreme old age, Dr. Alzheimer was perplexed. Why should a middle-aged woman be suffering from the effects of old age? Her condition continued to deteriorate while she was at the clinic and ultimately, she was reduced to what could be called a vegetative state. Four and a half years later when the woman died, Dr. Alzheimer was anxious to examine her brain. Looking through a newly invented microscope at stained slices of her cortex, the doctor discovered a disturbing phenomenon. Lumps of plaque and tangled bundles of fibrils had strangled the neurons that normally operate as message carriers in the brain.[105] The neurons and the neurotransmitters, chemicals that send messages to cells, are responsible for everything from walking and talking to memory.[106] The neurons were so compromised by debris that they were unable to operate. This gluing up is generally thought to begin in the hippocampus (the area of the brain controlling emotions, learning and short term memory) and moves on from there until many parts of the brain are affected.[107]

This altered condition of the brain reminded Virginia of a spark plug trying to fire. The poor spark plug sputters and spurts away, but a lot of built up gunk sadly prevents it from doing its job. It never produces a good enough spark, so the engine doesn't fire. Although lack of maintenance was probably responsible for the poor performance of the spark plug, this is where the analogy ends. The cause of the strange physiological occurrence now named after Dr. Alzheimer has, as of yet, not been determined. A disturbing statistic reports, after the age of eighty-five there is a fifty percent chance of developing Alzheimer's disease. [108]   There is no cure, but some medications seem to slow down the process.[109] However, slowing down the process is only treating the symptoms.[110] A vaccine to stop plaque formation may be in the works but plaques may not be the only problem. There are a lot of *buts*.

When Virginia's children were newborn, she would watch them lying in the crib waving their arms and legs in the air. At first all their movements were reflexes; not done on command.[112] As the brain matured and their eyes began to focus, between two and eight months old,[113] they began to notice they could make their hands and fingers move. Although the fetus can move its hands and legs and touch its face and body while in the womb, it is not until after birth that the visual cortex is stimulated by light.[114] *What an amazing realization it is that these strange looking appendages are part of me and I can make them move!* After a short time of moving fingers and toes and putting them in the mouth, the girls would fall into a deep sleep. Working out how to make things move is exhausting. Not physical work but brain work. A baby is born with no skills. Everything he or she does is learned. It is a gradual process, building up over the first years of life. Soon, the toddler is copying his elders, walking and talking; skills are learned and memories are built.[115]

An educator once described the learning process to Virginia in terms of a field of new grass. The first time crossing the field leaves no impression. The next time on the same path might bend a few blades. After many crossings along the path, the grass starts to wear down and the path becomes visible. In a similar way, the neural circuits (the paths) in the brain create learned patterns. The pathways become memories called "engrams."[116] Damage to the brain can compromise the path. When a person suffers damage from an accident or stroke, it is like a huge boulder falling in the middle of the field. Some of the paths are obstructed, the messages cannot pass and the neurons become starved of nutrients and die. Sometimes, depending on the degree of damage, the clever brain can find new paths around the boulder, but it takes time and hard work.[117] The amazing brain is continually changing, processing and modifying ("cognitive restructuring") itself with each new piece of input.[118] New neurons can be generated to replace the dying ones and new pathways created.[119] Diligence and repetition are required to create the new paths, but it can be done.[120] This was the challenge faced by Virginia's daughter after her surgery. She persevered in search of improved function, trying many different therapies and strategies. One of these was Taub Therapy developed by Dr. Edward Taub at the University of Alabama. This therapy is designed for brain injury patients and is based on the theory of Constraint-Induced Movement

Therapy.[121] The unaffected limb is constrained and the affected limb is forced to take on tasks. The brain is rewired to improve the function of the affected limb. During the therapy Nicola had amazing changes which have continued to materialize long since the program.

When Alzheimer's disease strikes, the situation is different from an accident or stroke. The gradual gluing up of the brain begins and the result is an equally gradual *unlearning* of all we have so carefully stored during a lifetime.[122] Loss of short-term memory comes first, followed by loss of recognition of familiar people, places and things, initially manifested as episodes of total confusion. Curiously, the memory controlled by the hippocampus is the area to develop last in an infant. Alzheimer's reverses the learning process.[123] Later, words are lost as well as control of movement and bodily functions. It is as though the person is returning to the womb and total dependency.[124] The brain/body connection seems to be lost. With Alzheimer's disease, it is as though a bucket of sludge has been poured down the middle of the field. As we try to cross the paths, the sludge gets spread around even more. The grass becomes matted and things become even stickier. Eventually, we cannot cross at all. We're just stuck in the muck.

Other factors, such as environmental or substance impact, can create symptoms similar to dementia. Symptoms of other related diseases such as Parkinson's disease, Creutzfeldt-Jakob disease, Diffuse Lewy Body disease or Pick's disease can be confused with Alzheimer's, but they are not the same. The correct diagnosis and treatment plan is essential.[125] Normal aging also affects the hippocampus, which is responsible for short-term memory, and creates similar physiology in the brain, but not to such an extent as Alzheimer's. It is, therefore, easy to confuse early signs of Alzheimer's with normal aging and vice versa.[126]

Alzheimer's seems to strike later in life and Virginia ran across quite a few clients who had been diagnosed with it. Although her mother had dementia, it was not considered to be Alzheimer's. Alice became forgetful and confused but did not completely lose her body/brain connection as later stage Alzheimer's patients tend to do. She had a vascular dementia caused by numerous small strokes. Her symptoms were similar but not progressive. However, as with the Alzheimer's sufferers, she felt lost, confused and abandoned.

Over the years Virginia noticed some unusual commonalities among her clients with Alzheimer's. Many of them had created giant barriers against anyone and everyone, regardless of the relationship. This seemed to start early on as they became aware of their symptoms. They began with denial, refusing to accept the symptoms, both to others and to themselves.[127] The problem may have been exacerbated by the failure of caregivers to seek professional help because the problems were dismissed as signs of normal aging.[128]

As the disease progresses, the barriers become larger, sometimes almost insurmountable. It is as if the person no longer trusts him or herself, especially the mind, and that mistrust translates to everyone around. It is founded in fear and no amount of talking can dispel it. This mistrust creates a difficult situation for family and caregivers. The sufferer gets angry, sometimes violent, feels everyone is against him or her and ultimately retreats into him or herself.[129] When Alice was a resident at the assisted living facility in Florida a couple lived in the apartment next door. The husband suffered from Alzheimer's. He had gotten to the point where he did not always recognize his wife and sometimes thought she was a stranger. They both would have faired better if professional staff had cared for him, but it was hard for his wife to let go. They had been married for so many years; she could not come to terms with losing him like this. One day, she had gone out shopping and, when she returned home, she let herself in with her key. Her husband mistook her for an intruder and, grabbing a lamp, hit her on the head. Unfortunately, her injuries were fatal. Alice called Virginia to announce there had been a murder in her building.

The husband and wife described above had lost their connection and were no longer able to communicate. Visual and auditory exchanges are usual means of communication. When Virginia is mad at one of her daughters, she might raise her voice, in person or on the phone. In person, the daughter sees her mother's anger as well as hearing it. On the phone, it is only her voice. In both instances Virginia's energy and emotions are also evident.

Talking on the phone to someone with dementia is usually not very satisfactory. Virginia recalled her mother had difficulty following a conversation on the phone and Alice would often hang up out of frustration. An Alzheimer's patient might listen for while and then look around for someone to explain what is going on. A face-to-face conversation is likely to be more productive. That, too, can prove to be difficult. First, the visual recognition may be impaired. When she approached Allison, Virginia would be greeted by a blank stare. Allison's vision was compromised. Although her eyesight was most likely intact, her brain did not understand the image and she did not register what she was seeing. She may have recognized Virginia as a person but the meaning seemingly ended there.

Second, auditory recognition may be compromised. When speaking directly to Allison, she may or may not understand what is being said. She may respond because she recognizes it as speech and her brain may register some of the words but probably not all of them. The brain also has to connect the words and make sense of them. This type of connection can become impaired fairly early. The level of recognition and communication can remain the same for a long period, years even, and then suddenly, there will be a noticeable shift. The Alzheimer's Association has a list of progressive stages of the disease.[130] What we often do not appreciate is, in the late stages when the visual and auditory levels are compromised or possibly absent altogether, the other levels of the individual, the emotions and energy, are still intact. This is where communication and connection can still occur. Even if a loved one does not recognize you by sight or by your voice, he or she will always recognize your touch.

Virginia met Mollie when her husband requested massage for her. Mollie had been a resident of the care facility for a few months. She had been diagnosed with Alzheimer's disease but otherwise had no serious health problems. On the first visit Virginia found her sitting on a sofa in the lounge with her walker positioned in front of her. She was unable to rise on her own, but the walker was there in case she needed it. If anyone tried to move it away they were immediately reminded that it belonged where it was. Mollie had a stern look about her with a set jaw, which instantly brought back memories of Grandmother Kress. She stared straight ahead. Virginia sat next to her, introduced herself and gently placed her hand on Mollie's arm. She asked if Mollie would like a massage. Foolish question, she soon discovered. Without looking at Virginia, Mollie replied she would not care for a massage at the moment and that she did not like to be fussed with.

A few days later, Virginia went looking for Mollie again. Sitting next to her as before and, having learned her lesson the last time, she asked Mollie if she could give her a back rub. Mollie thought she was supposed to be going somewhere but as it would only take a few minutes, she agreed and managed a weak smile. Touching her shoulder, Virginia felt her tense up. It was an easy jump to the conclusion that Mollie was not used to being touched, especially by strangers. Whatever emotions she may have had were well hidden behind a stern countenance. After about five minutes, she said she had had enough.

Don't waste your time on me, she added. *It's hardly a waste of my time,* Virginia countered. *I am enjoying being with you.* Mollie again smiled weakly and continued to stare straight ahead. After a few minutes, the entire conversation was replayed. This time, Virginia stopped and said she would see her later.

This type of encounter continued for a few months. Virginia persevered until, one day, she placed her hands on Mollie's shoulders, and Mollie responded broad smile and asked Virginia how she had been. Suddenly she recognized the touch. This was a breakthrough! From then on the sessions with Mollie were more rewarding. She was pleased when Virginia came to see her and responded as though greeting an old friend. One day Mollie was sitting near the nurses' station in a high-backed chair with arms. Virginia knelt next to her and held her hand. *You're so cute. Stand up and let me see your suit,* Mollie commanded. Virginia obliged. She gently started to rub Mollie's back and shoulders, waiting for her body to respond. All the time they talked about what Mollie had been doing. The conversation was vague and out of some time in her past. Generally, Virginia agreed and backed up anything Mollie said. The conversation became confused as the time frame, location and players jumped around like a pop corn machine with two other residents in nearby wheelchairs chiming in from time to time. Virginia maintained physical contact with Mollie the entire time.

On another occasion, Virginia found Mollie in the activities room participating in the "bounce the big green ball" activity. The nurse appeared asking if she could interrupt long enough to give Mollie some medication for the fungus under her nails. After the nurse finished Virginia sat next to Mollie so they could chat about her morning, which had been uneventful, while Virginia gently worked on her back and arms. *I want to kiss you*, Mollie repeated several times, to which Virginia obliged. They returned to the ball bouncing session and Mollie bounced the ball back to the aide more vigorously than anyone else.

On the next visit, Mollie was again sitting in a chair near the nurses' station with her walker in front of her. She was conversing with Jane, a long time resident who was sitting in her wheel chair on Mollie's left. As Virginia approached, Mollie smiled and said to Jane, *Isn't she cute?* Virginia sat on the table on Mollie's right side so as not to disturb her relationship with Jane who seemed to have changed very little over the years. She had always been in a wheelchair and she had always been dissatisfied with her accommodations. Virginia began to lightly stroke Mollie's shoulder. *What have you been doing?* Mollie initiated. Her question sparked a rather disjointed conversation with Jane who said she was waiting to go home when her son came to pick her up. Mollie said she had been working that morning and was looking forward to a rest. Virginia continued to work on her back and neck and on her arms and hands which were very elegant. Mollie had long fingers which would be perfect to model jewelry or gloves on TV. Each of these sessions lasted only fifteen minutes which may sound brief but is enough at one time. Frequency is the most important factor and repeated short visits are more beneficial than an isolated long one.

More recently, when Virginia arrived at the facility, she found Mollie sitting in a chair, staring straight ahead. During an activity, she sat quietly, not participating. Virginia walked past her but there was no sign of recognition until she touched Mollie's shoulder when she began to glow like a candle as she realized it was someone she knew, although each time Virginia took on a different persona from her past. She became very animated and a lot of laughter over something ensued. The care facility had one of those PA systems that loudly announced messages and phone calls for the staff. It would irritate most people to have these blaring announcements in their residence but Mollie had worked in a hospital setting during an earlier period of her life and the quality of sound coming from the PA system was familiar to her, reassuring and comforting.

Over the years, Virginia noticed her conversations with Mollie became increasingly disjointed. She went through a period of great anxiety about something in her past. As they talked about it, Virginia could feel Mollie's shoulders relax under the light touch and by the end of the session she was laughing. They agreed there was nothing to be done and she could stop worrying. Most of the time Virginia had no idea what was upsetting her and she was not capable of verbalizing the exact problem. It didn't matter. The gentle touch and reassurance that she was not alone was all she needed. This same session repeated for several months until it gradually passed and Mollie became more content. In fact, she was delighted when Virginia arrived and invariably requested a kiss. It seemed that she placed Virginia as someone she knew and trusted, through her emotion and energy. Sometimes she says, *Don't forget me.* As if Virginia could forget her!

As Alzheimer's disease progresses to the point where the body is severely compromised, communication, as we normally know it, is lost. During the day, Gerald sat in his wheelchair either in his room, in the hallway or in one of the common rooms. He did not register visual images or sounds, but he was very angry. His neck and shoulders were taut and stiff and he grasped the tray attached to the chair in front of him. With one fist he banged on the tray and rocked back and forth. He continually yelled loudly, not words, just noise. When Virginia touched him, he didn't seem to notice. She waited with her hands on his shoulders and back. His energy was strong, as was his anger. Virginia had a great deal of difficulty getting through his distress. Sometimes knowing a little background can be helpful, sometimes it can be misleading. The family members may have an idea about what is distressing their loved one or they may be way off base. If she was unable to get through to a client, Virginia might ask the family for some history and, in Gerald's case, she decided some input from the family could help. She spoke with a relative who informed her that a few years ago, Gerald's wife had passed away. At the time he had blamed a hospital error for her death and the family felt he was still carrying that anger. That small piece of information gave Virginia some insight about how to communicate with Gerald. During subsequent sessions, she focused her intention on his life with his beloved wife and on letting go of his anger. She could feel his energy resisting the idea. One day, after a couple of months, she felt a sudden release in his energy. It seemed that he was able to let go of his anger and he became calmer and stopped banging his chair. The anger may have been keeping him going.

Entering an Alzheimer's facility can be alarming for visitors. The unit is locked for the safety of the residents who might otherwise wander off. The images and sounds can be disturbing for visitors and even for the staff members who are there regularly. A group of people sitting in wheelchairs with no expression, looking upset, crying, shouting or moaning can be distressing to visitors. It is important to remember the residents do not see and hear the same things the visitor sees and hears.[131] Studies are underway to determine if agitation in people with dementia can be managed through the environment, for example, using light therapy.[132] Any reduction in discomfort is helpful however it can be difficult to tell how much the sufferer actually registers. For one thing, the deterioration varies from person to person and another misleading factor is that the level of recognition can come and go. At some stage, the people in wheelchairs appear to be just bodies. The cries and shouts are just noise for those in the later stages of the disease.[133] The brain does not register any of these things as disturbing and, finally, the brain doesn't register them at all. This is the progression of the disease. The only way to get a clue about how much the patient recognizes is by continued observation and continuous interaction; repeated visits. Visits can be short, as short as fifteen minutes since long visits can be tiring and ultimately distressing for the Alzheimer's patient. Frequent and brief is the key.[134]

There is hope however. Ultimately, the mind (as distinct from the brain), emotions, spirit and energy seem to remain intact and it is on these levels that we can continue to communicate and reassure the sufferer, enhancing the reduced quality of life. The question is how to make the connections on these levels. It is possible to connect with someone remotely, through thought and intention, prayer or energy, but by far the easiest and most powerful way is through touch. All the other levels can be reached when hands are touching the body. The Alzheimer's patients respond to touch but for the visitor it is a matter of recognizing the response. Much research has been done on the effects of touch on premature babies and infants. The resounding conclusion is that without touch, the baby does not thrive and grow into a confident adult.[135] Touch sends the message of self-worth.[136] So it is with the dementia sufferer.[137]

By merely placing hands gently and lightly on the person's body, a connection can be established. By itself, massage will reduce the anxiety and depression associated with Alzheimer's[138] but including energy in the connection enhances the communication. With Alzheimer's patients, it seems to be more difficult to connect through the head, a usual connection point for some therapies. The stomach is sometimes called the second brain and is a good conduit as are the feet. Alzheimer's patients seem to set up barriers which can be overcome but it is invariably a matter of re-establishing trust. This takes time and repetition. The body begins to recognize the touch and, even if the brain doesn't recognize the person, the energy responds and a connection can be made on a deep level.

Consider Sandra who had been a resident at the care facility for a year or so. She sat in her wheelchair and fidgeted and tried to move around the room, using her feet to propel the chair. The staff would become quite irritated with her and usually tried to block her into a corner. She was generally cheerful but, in addition to not being able to walk, her verbal skills were failing resulting in few sentences and then a smile and a laugh. She loved having her back and shoulders rubbed and would often say, *That feels good.* Within a few years of visiting her twice a week, Virginia began to routinely find her lying in bed. Sandra had been diagnosed with Alzheimer's.

The bed was low so Virginia sat on the edge stroking her hair in slow motions and stopping just off her skull to assess the energy. The energy coming from her head was very low.

On one occasion, Sandra was in bed lying on her side so Virginia sat on the side of her bed. As with other Alzheimer's' patients that she had witnessed, Sandra's energy was displaced on the left side of her body so it was less intrusive to sit on her right side. Virginia had long since stopped trying to draw her energy back to the center of her body as it didn't stay there and seemed to have little effect. Sandra's eyes were open and she was relaxed. She smiled and nodded as Virginia stroked her head and spoke softly to her. Taking advantage of her position Virginia started placing her fingers gently along her spine. She slowly worked down the right side of Sandra's spine and back up the other side. Sandra became increasingly relaxed during this methodical procedure. She shakily reached up to grasp Virginia's hand. Her skin was very thin and she often had bruises on her wrists from struggling with the aides. She was a very private person and intensely disliked having her adult diaper changed. Virginia could always tell if an aide had just changed her because she would be lying in bed with her blanket firmly clutched under her chin. She would look away and it would take a few minutes before Virginia could get through to her.

Toward the end of her life, Sandra was suddenly taken to the hospital and, as her family lived a good distance away, Virginia followed her there. She was in the emergency room surrounded by a curtain and attended by a young doctor who was concerned that she did not respond to his questions. By that stage, Sandra had not spoken a word for several years. Sandra's body was tense, like a bowstring, possibly knowing she was in a strange place. Virginia approached the low cot and put one hand on her shoulder and the other on her stomach. She instantly relaxed. She even opened her eyes a crack and managed a tiny smile. *Amazing!* Her response reaffirmed Virginia's mission. It seemed Sandra recognized her touch and was relieved someone knew where she was. Even though Sandra had not been able to communicate visually or orally, she still connected with Virginia. It is as important for Alzheimer's sufferers as for others to know their lives have been witnessed. If there is such a thing as an average life span for an Alzheimer's patient, it is about eight to ten years after diagnosis but it can stretch out to as long as twenty years.[139] As the disease progresses and recognition is lost, touch remains the only means of contact and reassurance.

Chapter 7

The Field

Virginia knew energy had something to do with atoms jumping and jiggling around and when lots of atoms are put together in an organized structure, they make up what looks to us like a solid mass. A piece of furniture, a tree, the dog, all are made up of billions of atoms. All well and good! That is our reality. So what was this about energy?

During the many classes Virginia ultimately took with Harriet, from time to time Harriet would reference a man named Lansing Barrett Gresham. She had met him at a training, given by Moshe Feldenkrais,[140] many years ago and they had remained friends. Over the years, Lansing had developed a healing modality called Integrated Awareness® (IA)[141] and, at that time, had a center called Touchstone located in Cotati, California, north of San Francisco. In his new location in Rohnert Park, California, Lansing teaches workshops and classes as well as training and individual sessions. Virginia and Nicola decided to register for one of the weekend workshops so they could see for themselves what all the fuss was about. They drove up Highway 101 until they arrived in the town of Cotati, turned in at a sign saying Touchstone and located the office, only to be directed to the upstairs of a building across the parking lot. A large empty room greeted them but as they were a little early no one else was there. There were no chairs, so they sat down on the floor. They were getting used to the floor by now. Gradually people started filtering in, gathering and talking in small groups. They didn't know anyone so they sat by themselves at the side. Virginia was relieved to see people appearing from a closet carrying back-jacks – those canvas covered metal frames with a cushion that goes on the floor. She had encountered them at Esalen. They support the back and make the whole sitting on the floor experience much more comfortable. She rushed to grab a couple for Nicola and herself. They joined the second row of the semi-circle that was forming. A woman made a few announcements that meant nothing to Virginia and then, with precision timing, a tall graying man with a beard appeared and took up a position on a bar stool which had been placed in the center of the semi-circle. *That must be Lansing,* Virginia whispered to Nicola. He introduced himself and greeted a few people in the circle. Then he looked directly at Virginia and Nicola and asked if they had met before. After they had recovered from an attempt to melt into the floor, they responded together that, no, in fact, they had not met before. He asked why they had come. Silence. Eventually they blamed Harriet and that was good enough.

Lansing proceeded to talk to the group for about an hour and a half, but Virginia did not follow any of what he said. After the break the class divided up into groups of four. Back-jacks decamped and massage tables appeared out of other closets. Each group clustered around a table and Lansing started to give instructions. One person lying on the table was to imagine him or herself in a particular situation and the other three, with *hands on* (there's that expression again), were to help guide the subject through a process of self-discovery, perhaps healing. Phrases like "life purpose", "going inside", "being present", "showing up" and "karma" (what's that again?[142]) were uttered. Virginia didn't know if she was experiencing any of these things and she still had not the faintest idea what he was talking about and the answers to her questions only led to more questions. Confusion is good. It is to be expected, she was told. Clarity will come out of confusion. OK, hang in there.

The second day was similar to the first and by the end of the workshop, Virginia was aware she had experienced something, but she was not sure exactly what it was. She and Nicola drove home to think about it. After that experience, one would think Virginia would never venture back. Did she want to be confused? No, she had already felt confused at Buddha Camp, as her daughter's friend had insisted on calling it, but she did want to get to the bottom of what seemed like a bizarre modality, so she attended on a few more weekends. After many conversations and more strange experiences, Virginia began to get a glimpse of what Lansing was on about and, after a rocky start, she found the Integrated Awareness® community to be a dedicated and embracing group of people.

About the time Virginia was investigating Integrated Awareness,® she went with her daughter, Charlotte, on a trip to Southeast Asia, a part of the world she had never before visited. The pair first went to Australia to visit some friends who had there from London. They then flew back to Bangkok and on to Katmandu. Virginia was scheduled to leave on a trek in the vicinity of Annapurna, but the day before the departure, her small group was informed that there would be a public strike and demonstration on the following day. Not only was their departure postponed, but also they were advised not to leave the hotel that day. It was nice to sleep in and then to sit in the garden under the white stupa[143] stained with yellow saffron. A high white wall protected the garden from what turned out to be a little street violence. An employee of the hotel announced that an important yogi would be giving a special class in the afternoon. Yoga sounded good. Virginia had spent a few years practicing yoga, mostly because everyone said it was good for you. Yoga had been quite a fad a few years ago. It was still very popular, Virginia thought, but she hadn't been going to classes lately. She felt good about it when she did go, more limber and it felt good to stretch. The "Salute to the Sun"[144] was a good, all-around exercise. At least it was something she knew, so, with the support of two other ladies in her group, she went along. It was a small room, crowded with quite a few people who also had been told not to leave the hotel. Virginia found a mat and sat down cross-legged. Luckily, the yogi had a good command of the English language because her Nepali was lacking. He demonstrated a pose and started talking about the effects of the pose on the digestive system. Then he moved on to muscle relaxation. Toward the end, the familiar Salute to the Sun showed up, but the whole encounter was quite different from what Virginia had previously experienced. This practice of yoga was intended to sustain or restore balance and good health to the body. The poses helped the body to move the energy where it had become depleted. There was so much more to this practice than the exercise she remembered. She flew back to the US to attend another IA® workshop with new information and a new curiosity.

There are several theories about the existence of the individual. Nearly all of them agree that a person exists on more than one level and the body, which we know and love sometimes, is only one of them.[145] In IA,® Lansing divides us into five levels of consciousness. After the body, the spirit is another obvious level, as is emotion. He also regards the mind as a level which not in the physiological realm and therefore separate from the brain (the brain belongs to the body; it is physical).[146] Finally, there is energy. All living things, plants included, are surrounded by electro-magnetic energy. Kirlian photography claims to record this energy on film, however the results are controversial.[147] This energy is sometimes termed a *field* of energy because, or so Virginia thought, for each entity, the field has finite borders, like a field of wheat, with the physical body sitting in the middle. That explanation sounded good at the time. Virginia was to find out later that it was somewhat more complex than that.

The energy in question continually circulates through and around the body. In Eastern modalities it is sometimes called the aura. The energy field can extend out, many feet, around the person. Have you ever walked down the street and had a prickly feeling that someone was following you, perhaps to do you harm? That *sixth sense* was your energy field noticing the energy from someone near you. The ideal state for the human being, again according to Lansing, is for all the levels (physical body, mind, emotion, energy and spirit) to be congruent with each other. To do so, all parts must be present in the here and now. Some of this reminded Virginia of her experiences at the Buddhist retreat. Encouraging mindfulness, in other words, living in the present, was a common theme.[148] *How many times,* Virginia mused, *have I gotten in my car to drive home, only to arrive on the doorstep without any recollection of how I got there? I have read a page of a book only to realize I had no recollection of what I read and had to read it again.*[149] Her mind, and perhaps other levels as well, had not been congruent with her body, an all too common occurrence.[150] Only when we are present and whole, and with a clear intention about where we are and what we are doing, can we truly heal.[151] Exploring the human condition for each individual, and looking for ways in which the individual can reach the best possible state, seems to be the mantra of Integrated Awareness.®

Energy is one of Lansing's levels and Virginia had encountered the idea before in other settings. It is a complex subject – more complex than she had ever imagined. There are many theories about energy, sometimes called "the energetic body", but they all have things in common. For example, Therapeutic Touch (TT) "is used to balance and promote the flow of human energy. . . [It] has a substantial base of formal and clinical research. This research has shown TT is useful in reducing pain, improving wound healing, aiding relaxation, and easing the dying process."[152]

In massage school, one of the modalities Virginia studied was Shiatsu, a form of massage originating in Japan. Different from the Swedish massage more common in the West, Shiatsu aims at aligning or reorganizing the body's energy in order to promote good health. Similarly, in Traditional Chinese Medicine (TCM), there are both *universal energy* and *vital energy*. Universal energy comes from the earth (*yin*, female) and from the sky (*yang*, male)[153] and is available for anyone who needs it. Vital energy is the energy belonging to an individual. It is the life force or the will to live. Without vital energy, there is no life.[154] Together they make up cosmic bio-energy called *chi*,[155] (also spelled ch'i or qi,)[156] or *prana*, depending on where you are in the world. Back in China, there are several sources of chi: *original chi* is the energy you were born with, given to you by your parents; *nutritional chi* comes from the food you eat; *air chi* comes from the air you breathe.[157] The latter, along with *earth and sky (solar) chi*, are all acquired chi, which is used up and then renewed. Original chi belongs to you alone and is used up little by little over a lifetime.[158] The breath is closely associated with chi because it is through breathing that we can feel the energy entering the body. [159]

According to TCM, the yin and yang energies (chi) run smoothly around small and large circuits in the body on predetermined pathways and in a predetermined direction. Only when yin and yang are in perfect balance is the chi strong. When they are out of balance, the body is vulnerable. It is the combination of the circulation of chi and the circulation of blood that is responsible for a healthy body. The pathways, or circuits, of the continuously circulating chi are called meridians and it is on the meridians that acupuncture and acupressure find the points where they can help to rebalance yin and yang when there is illness so the body can *gain chi*.[160] Strong chi can ward off "pathogenic factors" leading to illness and disease.[161]

While acupuncture and herbal medicine are used to promote a restoration of good health, chi gong (also chi kung) and massage, along with eating properly, are used to maintain health.[162] Many acupuncturists are also chi gong masters and use it for healing purposes as well. Chi gong is defined as "manipulation of vital energy."[163] It is an ancient form of Chinese healing in which the chi gong master has perfect control over his own chi and can use it externally to influence the chi of another.[164, 165] Based on control of vital energy, it is practiced off the body between two inches and a foot from the patient.[166] Chi gong can take a variety of forms. It can be similar to a martial art, quite physical with potentially serious consequences,[167] or it can take a much more quiet form. In any case, it requires control of breath, body and thoughts.[168] During Virginia's brief encounter with chi gong at Esalen, the class practiced breathing, movements and poses. She didn't have any feeling of control over her chi but, of course, she didn't really know what that would feel like, and later she thought it may have happened without her realizing it. It was curious she chose the workshop at random. She remembered simply being attracted to the description of the discipline.

For Virginia the most interesting thing about this healing form was that it occurs by way of a transfer or manipulation of energy from one person to another. The energy of the chi gong master acts to *fortify* the chi of the patient, thereby increasing the patient's "own ability to fight disease."[169] The evidence in China of the power of chi therapy, chi gong or acupuncture, is overwhelming. All are considered legitimate forms of treatment.[170]

From all of this, Virginia began to understand that vital energy can become depleted for a number of reasons such as illness or an accident. The dangers of low energy lie in vulnerability to disease and other invasive energies entering the aura and causing damage to the body, mind or spirit. Vital energy can be replaced or bumped up with universal energy, the general energy all around us. This can be done through self-discipline or with the aid of another. But the other does not have to be an expert chi gong master; it could be a caring party such as a family member. Presence and intention alone can be healing.[171]

Intention? Virginia was told, by her teachers, that it was possible to influence energy through her intention by drawing universal energy into her field or by having it channeled it into her field by another individual, thus restoring her energy. If she intended for energy to move, it would. This also meant she could channel universal energy to others by simply announcing to herself it would happen. This sounded a little suspect to her, especially since she wasn't sure this energy actually existed. After all, she couldn't see it or feel it! She needed proof. The proof came in the form of a workshop with Dr. Mary Clark.

Virginia first met Mary Clark at Harriet's where they were attending the same workshop. Mary's descriptions of prana were intriguing. Virginia understood prana to be another name for chi, only originating in the ayurvedic (Indian or Hindu) tradition. She ultimately attended a workshop conducted by Dr. Clark at the California Institute for Human Science in Encinitas, California. Mary teaches a variety of beginning and advanced Pranic Healing classes which focus on healing and repairing the energy field, the one Virginia couldn't see or feel. It is the very interaction between the energy body and the physical body that forms the basis of pranic healing.[172] Like chi gong, all the therapy is done in the field without touching the body. Everyone knows what it feels like to be coming down with a cold. The theory is, the cold is lurking in your energy field outside the physical body and, if it can be cleared from your energy field, your body will not be affected.

Virginia was assured it is possible to learn how to see the energy surrounding living things. Mary first took them outside to look at a stand of trees on the horizon. Trees, being large, have large energy fields. As they squinted their eyes and stared at the trees, everyone in the class, without exception, was able to discern a hazy shimmering surrounding the distant trees. That shimmering was the energy field. Virginia was fascinated once she realized she could see it. Prana comes from the sun (solar prana), the air (ozone prana) and the earth (ground prana).[173]

Sounds familiar. As they discovered in the practice sessions, the quality of the prana takes on a different appearance according to the state of the person. If the person is injured, it might seem cloudy. If the person is upset, it appears agitated. If the person is happy, it looks sleek and smooth. The field, or aura, might contain colors which reflect different physical and psychological states of the individual. Blue is associated with spirituality, pink reflects love and compassion, red is pain or anger, etc.

The group trooped back into the classroom to pair up and using one hand, palm open, slowly moved that hand closer to their partner's body. *When you feel a kind of barrier, stop,* they were told. Virginia found it helped to close her eyes. Sure enough, she did feel a kind of bump, like the quality of the air had changed. She opened her eyes to find her hand about twelve inches away from her partner's shoulder. The energy can extend several feet out from the body in layers: the closer to the body, the more dense the layer. It is the inside layer that is the most visible and also the one she could feel. She was convinced.

It seems there can be holes in the energy field caused by any number of things, such as illness or an accident or even caused by internal emotional problems.[174] The holes allow for unwanted energy to creep in and further disturb the field. Problems can also occur due to blocks in energy circulation. The blocks prevent the vital energy from flowing smoothly through the body reaching all the body parts. Like holes, they upset the field and allow for disturbances, such as pathogens or dysfunctions in the field which lead to disease or illness, but can be healed with new prana.[175] Using his *intention*, the pranic healer directs prana to the patient who then can use the new energy in the healing process.[176] The healer focuses on chakras, which are energy centers lined up vertically along the center of the bio-plasmic body, the invisible energy body. Starting at the base of the spine, the first chakra links us to the earth for support and the seventh, the crown chakra located on top of the head, links us to the universe and the Devine.[177]

Smaller chakras are located on other parts of the body. On the part of the patient, a positive attitude is useful for the healing to take place. Daily affirmations are encouraged.[178] It is not necessary to have any special powers to practice pranic healing.[179] Anyone can learn it. Virginia was relieved to hear that since she was certain that she did not possess special powers.

During her daughter's rehabilitation, Virginia accompanied her on a visit to a new therapist who had been recommended for her condition. Virginia had recently come from the workshop about energy therapy so, at the time, she was particularly attuned to it. She was practicing. It was like having a new toy. She couldn't help watching to see what was going on in people's energy fields. On this occasion, they were shown into the therapist's room. Nicola sat on the therapy table and Virginia sat in a chair on one side waiting for the therapist who came in, asked some questions and then began working with Nicola. Virginia pulled her chair away from the table and sat quietly observing. She noticed immediately that the therapist had what she liked to call *busy* energy. Although her outward demeanor was calm and professional at all times, her energy field appeared to be agitated. The hour-long session ended and the therapist left the room. Nicola took a few minutes to get up and when they went out to the desk, Virginia asked the receptionist if she could ask the therapist a question. The receptionist replied: *Oh, she had to leave. She was in an automobile accident on her way here and she had to go to see about her car. That explains it,* Virginia thought. Of course her energy was agitated after a car accident which is distressing for anyone. *My energy would have been upset, too.* Our energy reflects our true state even though we may not be completely conscious of it.

Her experience with Pranic Healing led Virginia to be more attuned to conversations about energy and fields. She began to hear references to energy from people who were not talking about the ancient Asian systems based on chi or prana, meridians or chakras. One of these people was Dr.

Peter Levine. He and a colleague, Dr. Maggie Phillips, were conducting a weekend workshop concentrating on healing following trauma. *Brain surgery is pretty traumatic,* Virginia reasoned, so she and Nicola decided to attend. They headed back along the beautiful Pacific coast to Big Sur.

A group of about twenty people gathered in the Big Yurt, a large cream colored canvas teepee, at Esalen. The light filtered through a hole in the center of the roof in a glittering shaft giving the environment an ethereal atmosphere. They went around in a circle with the usual introductions. Dr. Levine presented himself and the ideas that developed into his trauma therapy, Somatic Experiencing (SE). Dr. Levine's approach to the individual reminded Virginia of Lansing. He described people as organisms made up of different parts: body, mind, instincts, intellect, emotions and spirituality all blending together to make the whole. His approach was holistic; no parts operate independently; only through all of the parts do we get a true sense of self.[180]

The discussion turned to trauma and animals' (including human) responses to life-threatening danger. The fight or flight response is common enough and its opposite, Herbert Benson's relaxation response, invokes a calming sense of well-being that can be healing.[181] Levine takes it further to a not-so-well-known response termed "immobility" or "freezing" in which the animal feigns death and enters an altered state of consciousness.[182] An example of this is a cheetah chasing an impala. When the impala senses the chase is over, it falls to the ground in a non-conscious state. In that state, the impala gives off minimal signals: no movement, little breath and low energy. The cheetah might bypass it altogether, not even seeing it, and the impala could get up and go on unharmed. On the other hand, should the cheetah find the animal, the impala would not feel the pain of death in the jaws of its predator.

Humans, in the face of a trauma, often choose not to react in this instinctual way, even though, in terms of recovery, it might be more favorable. This second-guessing of our animal instincts leaves us vulnerable to the effects of consciously experiencing a trauma[183] and subsequent traumatic stress brought on by the energy of the chase trapped in our bodies with no where to go.[184] More recent research has shown that trauma memory, which has become "locked in the nervous system . . . can become reactivated at the slightest reminder of the original trauma."[185] This could come from words, sounds, smells or any sensory input that could vaguely be associated with the event. In essence, the emotional connection to the trauma can filter down in the system to the body and get stuck there in the form of illness.[186] Releasing the trapped energy can be most helpful in avoiding adverse physiological effects.

At the workshop, armed with the impala analogy, the group divided up into pairs or threes. Virginia and Nicola were joined by a gray haired man whom they had never before met. By this time, they were used to working with total strangers and they proceeded to follow directions. The usual massage tables appeared and one person was elected to be on the table. Nicola went first, as she had a lot to say about trauma. Nicola was to imagine a happy place, where she felt safe and secure, and take a physical posture representing that feeling. Much of the approach was based on energy psychology which is a broad term covering different techniques. Among them are thought field therapy (TFT), eye movement desensitization and reprocessing (EMDR), ego-state therapy (Gestalt, psychosynthesis, neurolinguistic programming (NLP), transactional analysis), imagery, hypnosis and to name a few.[187] Whichever approach is taken, the overall goal is to obtain integrative results, the process affecting the whole person.[188] This is Somatic Experiencing (SE).

The gentleman and Virginia were to put their hands on (by now you know what that means) Nicola, wherever they were drawn. Next, the person on the table was to imagine a not-too-traumatic situation in their past. The therapists were to monitor the changes in the physical body as the person moved from the happy place to the threatened place. Ultimately, the goal was to find a place in the middle so the energy locked in the threatened place could be released. The healing, of course, was coming from within Nicola with Virginia and the man acting as guides and witnesses. Nicola was not trying to re-live the traumatic events, which could be painful, but was finding the symptoms of the past and putting them to rest.[189] At the end of the session, Virginia was excited to see her daughter able to flex her left foot more than she could at the start. The energetic shift in one area of the person forces the rest of the system to also shift.[190] That was the beginning of healing the trauma.

The touch component seemed to add to the release process and Dr. Phillips also reported achieving good results using collaborative efforts with body workers.[191] The whole experience was uplifting. Virginia and Nicola went home with a new understanding of the power of energy in the body and how it could be managed. It also served to convince Virginia even more that energy was real. It was not just made up as an answer to some question. Later she wondered if the brain forms the plaques associated with Alzheimer's disease as a defense mechanism so that the person does not have to continually relive a trauma. Maybe, once the brain realizes that it can block a bad experience, it gets carried away and begins to block all sorts of things! If the trauma had been released from the system, would the disease ever develop?

An important common factor of the Eastern energy practices is the concept and "awareness of the unity and mutual interrelation of all things and events."[192] The energy Virginia could see and feel, or at least she thought she could, was exciting but, in Western terms, chi had not been subject to scientific proof. To the Western scientist the body functions using peptides (a type of amino acid) to communicate with receptors all through the body and their actions are a manifestation of our emotions in physical terms. However there exists a small problem, that of energetic activity, which biochemistry cannot explain.[193] Energy in Western science falls into the category of physics. In high school, Virginia had a very serious physics teacher with unfortunate teeth that were hard to ignore. Although his neglected teeth were her main memory of him, she also remembered he was the teacher with the most passion about his subject. In class they drew vectors to indicate force, produced prisms to refract light and dropped objects on the floor to demonstrate gravity. Much of what they learned in the class seemed to be very practical and kind of obvious, but there were some unanswered questions: *Who says that Force equals mass times acceleration?* Sir Isaac Newton. *How did he know?* It was *proven* through repeated observations and experiments. It's Newton's Second Law of Motion. *What if he was wrong?* He wasn't.

Several decades later, a physicist named Alfonso Rueda mathematically proved that Newton's theory was correct.[194] Rueda's calculations incorporated the curious subject called quantum physics, which attempts to explain the characteristics of quanta (sub-atomic micro units of energy, the smallest of the small). This explanation turns out to be difficult. For one thing, both the momentum and the position of quanta cannot be determined at the same time because if quanta are moving, they are not fixed and if they are fixed, they are not moving.[195] Second, quanta sometimes behave like particles and sometimes like waves, depending upon whether or not someone is watching them (Wave-Particle Duality). This means everything is a collection of energetic waves until you observe them. Then, they turn into particles which are visible.[196] The entire universe and beyond is a huge *field* filled with quanta and, as they move through the field, they are constantly running into other quanta and each encounter is forever remembered.[197] According to the *non-locality* theory, an electron can communicate with another particle at any distance, even if there is no exchange of energy.[198] It is thought by some that the waves are composed of light pulses (biophotons) emitted by electrons, thus enabling molecules to communicate with each other.[199] When waves run into each other, they form a larger, more powerful wave creating an interaction called constructive interference. If they cross when one wave is at the top and the other is at the bottom of the pattern, both waves are lost (destructive interference).[200, 201] In fact, the field is nothing but moving, jiggling, shimmering bits of energy, all constantly interacting with each other.

The energy is not only in the particles but also in the gaps between the particles extending throughout the universe and beyond. Energy therefore is not a continuous stream, but is broken down into infinitesimally small pieces[202] and together they make up the field. It is sometimes called zero-point field or a sea of zero-point energy (or the electromagnetic quantum vacuum), because when all factors, such as matter or temperature, have been reduced to absolute zero, there is still energy present.[203] *This is beginning to sound a lot like Chinese universal energy.* Its existence explains why an electron doesn't lose its energy and die. In terms of quantum physics, the electron does give off energy, but it also takes energy back from the universal field.[204] Everything, even a void, is always buzzing with energy and therefore, there is a constant exchange of energy and information throughout the universe. These exchanges are on a sub-atomic level.

An example of two metal plates placed face-to-face, but not touching, seems to come up regularly in quantum discussions: the field between them is compressed and has greater density than the field surrounding them. Therefore, the attraction between them is increased. This is called the Casmir force.[205] Virginia wondered if this explained what happened when she approached another person with her hand to *feel* the aura or when she passed someone walking down the street and felt their presence. The compressed energy alerted her to the presence of the other person. Of course, she must be present in her body and aware of the situation. With her thoughts on something else, she could easily walk into a wall without noticing - until the bump. Buddhists spend time in sitting or walking meditation, allowing outside influences to come and go but staying present in their body. When you are present, you notice the energy of others because of the constant interaction in the fields. Virginia thought this idea explained why she could see the disturbed energy of her daughter's therapist after her automobile accident.

The Eastern ideas of chi and Western ideas of the field looked similar to Virginia. The field makes up her cells and the cells of everyone else. In the body, Eastern practices access energy through the meridians or chakras where energy is most concentrated, but there is also evidence that energy travels through connective tissue to other parts of the body.[206] Communication between life forms on the sub-atomic level is a result of a collective consciousness or universal consciousness.[207] What goes on in Virginia's cells can be felt by anyone with whom she has had an exchange. Both Eastern and Western ideas express the concept of the *whole* as unifying everything and everyone,[208] so, if there is a universal consciousness, then the energy in your field can be affected by the energy of others around you.[209] How are we affected by other people's energy? - positively or negatively, to different degrees, or not at all. Have you ever walked into a room full of people and suddenly found yourself in a bad mood for no particular reason? Or, suddenly found yourself in a good mood, again for no reason? The chances are you have been affected by the energy of someone around you. It follows that your energy can affect other living things just as much. Since trees and plants have energy fields too, it turns out those wacky-sounding people, who talk to their plants, are not so crazy after all. Sending loving and encouraging energy to your plants will nourish them and help them flourish.[210, 211] It works for people in the same way. Children provide the best example. An infant knows when Mom or Dad is in a bad mood and there is a lot of talk about the effects of encouragement and discouragement on children. Young children may be unable to comprehend adult reasoning, but they are certainly affected not only by body language and tone of voice, but also by energy.[212] If something is going on with parents or teachers, even if they outwardly appear to be calm and in control, the child will still pick up a disturbance in their field. Children are particularly vulnerable to the energy around them because until the age of about five, they operate in an alpha state.[213] They are growing, learning and absorbing all that is around them, good and bad.

Many adults, on the other hand, have devised numerous defense mechanisms to shield themselves from bad energy and also protect their own energy. Sometimes, this is a conscious effort and sometimes not. If universal energy is moving around and through us all the time, it seems plausible we can be aware of that energy if we pay attention to it. The person with the most organized energy (the more congruent or healthy) can influence the energy of someone who is ill with disorganized energy.[214] For any energy exchange to take place between two or more people, both must be available and open to the possibility so their fields can be synchronized.[215]

Some people are emotionally deprived and seem to be very needy. Needy people absorb energy. Virginia soon learned to recognize people who absorb available energy. They gave her all kinds of information about themselves that she really didn't need to know and they also often had many problems, usually with other people, requiring her advice. By the end of the conversation, she felt completely drained and exhausted. Chi gong masters are known to feel depleted following a healing exercise because they have given up some of their energy.[216] Virginia learned to hang onto her own vital energy merely through her intention by imagining a boundary, like a fence, around her that the other person could not cross, no matter what. That invisible boundary made it difficult for anyone to enter her field and take her energy.

Another technique used for self-protection is centering. When Virginia was a child she loved horseback riding. The instructor was always telling her to be centered. He meant she should have not only her weight, but also intention and focus, centered on the back of the animal. The horse could sense her control. When all the parts of your being are centered and focused in the present, it is difficult for others to invade your space uninvited.[217] In this way it is possible to create a boundary for yourself. A therapist may be a conduit for zero-point field or universal energy, an organizer for that energy, using it to help the other person if he or she needs it, without allowing the energy to disrupt his or her own field.[218]

The most important concept is there can be interaction between two or more people on levels other than the material (body) level. Mind, energy, emotion and spirit are all levels on which we can interact and talk to each other. The *talk* may not be in the familiar form of words but, nonetheless, it is a form of communication. It follows one could send healing thoughts through the field because we are all connected to each other through universal consciousness. Virginia's journey had unwittingly led her to this point, so let's see how these ideas showed up in practice.

Chapter 8

Strange Encounters

After all this discussion about energy work and the transfer of energy from one person to another and from the field, Virginia had one big question. It sounded like it could be happening, but how could she know for sure? How could she know it was happening to her or around her? She was still not entirely convinced that she believed any of it, but, if it was true, it was fascinating. She felt in danger of getting hooked.

In the CranioSacral Therapy II class, through the Upledger Institute, Virginia learned advanced techniques in using the craniosacral system as an indicator of the body's condition and responses. She couldn't help herself from signing up for the next class, SomatoEmotional Release I. The title itself was a mystery. Somato comes from somatics, in turn from the Greek word *soma*, which refers to the "living body." The soma is the internalized view of yourself, as opposed to what everyone else sees on the outside. It completes the *scientific* view of the person, that which is seen by another, to make a holistic approach to the human being. [219] The remainder of the course title, SomatoEmotional Release, seemed obvious. So this was going to be about letting go of any internal emotions that might be instigating physical problems and would, therefore, be better off discarded. How, as a therapist, to support the client in this process was the focus of the class.

There were two long weekend classes in this series and the first one Virginia could get into was back in the familiar Big Sur. Looking through the workbook, it appeared the class addressed connecting with the body's systems on a subconscious level. That again sounded familiar. There were techniques for locating and releasing energy cysts which could cause blockages in the system. There were vectors that could get out of alignment within the physical body. So, this was also working with energy. By that time, she was beginning to recognize some of the other participants and she felt less like an outsider. After the usual introductions, the instructor started to go through the workbook. There was a lot of waiting for the body to respond. This time, however, there might be dialogue between therapist and patient. The group was encouraged to look into the past for an event that had been distressing. Not everyone has had a life trauma but any unfortunate incident would do. In the next round, they recollected their parents and considered what their relationships had been with them. The class was sounding reminiscent of Dr. Levine's trauma workshop which Nicola and she had attended. Several times during the four days, people on the table would begin to sob. Something was certainly being released there!

For the second part of SomatoEmotional Release, Virginia traveled across the country to Washington D.C. The class was held in a large hotel like the class in San Francisco. There were other beginning courses going on at the same time which made Virginia feel important because she was now more advanced. It was a similar set up in a ballroom with tables and chairs and those same blue mats. There were about thirty people in the class. Things proceeded much like the last class with some new techniques to try. The big difference here was her response to the work. This was the first time that she had truly zoned out during a class. She was tired from traveling and staying in a hotel; she never slept as well as when she was at home. Virginia was the therapist and sat next to the table where Alica, her client, lay on her back on the blue mat. Virginia had one hand on Alica's abdomen and the other under her back. In the early afternoon after lunch - always a good time for a nap - Virginia thought she could fall asleep. She must have dozed off, or at least went into one of those altered states she kept hearing about but had never experienced. Kylea Taylor, in *The Ethics of Caring*, calls them "non-ordinary states of consciousness."[220] She was still aware of people around her, but she felt they were in another world. Or, maybe it was she who was in another world, or space, or time. It was hard to explain the feeling. She had her eyes closed when suddenly a large white egg appeared, floating in space. *What could that be?* She hadn't had eggs for breakfast or lunch. It had a luminous glow giving off a strange bluish-white light. She had no input into this scene except to observe it. When she came out of this strange state, she was still sitting in the same place and the teacher was talking. Although Virginia had been aware of him, she had not been listening. The session had ended and he was busy telling everyone to get feedback from his or her client. Alica told Virginia she had started to feel sad, especially toward the end of the session. Virginia described the egg and Alica started to cry. She had recently had a miscarriage and, not surprisingly, it had been preying on her mind. They decided the unborn child was all right because the egg was shining and appeared to be happy. They talked about her feelings a bit more and she said she felt better. Virginia was a little disturbed by this event, never having experienced anything like that before and didn't know what to make of it. The class ended and she returned to the west coast to think it over.

Some time later, Virginia was back at one of Lansing's workshops and this time she was on the table as the client. Perhaps she was tired again and seemed to fall asleep, but she remembered everything that went on the room. At one stage she had the distinct impression her body was rising from the table. Up and down she went several times, during which she saw her father with wings, until the episode ended and she lay back on the table. This time she was more disturbed than ever. Virginia asked Lansing what it meant and he said she was probably "approaching the hub." *What is that?* she wondered. The hub theory is a multiple lives theory in which each life is like a spoke extending from a wheel and it is possible to cross over the center and experience another life. This type of thing is possible in the quantum theory of non-locality where time and space, as we know them, do not exist.[221] Well, that was it for Virginia! What had she gotten herself into? If this was going to give her strange experiences, she was going back to her painting and other artwork which sounded much safer! She had started all this to help Nicola, but she hadn't bargained for this kind of encounter. When the class ended Virginia returned home and tried to put the whole incident behind her.

After a few days Virginia calmed down, but she was still resolved to give up this pursuit. It was all a little too strange. In a few weeks, Nicola and she were scheduled to go to Florida so her daughter could attend a two-week-long intensive workshop for brain and spinal cord injuries at the Upledger Institute. Everything was reserved and paid for, so she went along, far more skeptical than before. She would just support her daughter and maybe watch or maybe not. On the morning after their flight across the country, they arrived at the Institute a bit early. Outside stairs led to the office on the second floor of the gray wooden building, but no one was there so they waited in their rental car in the parking lot. Unlike California it was hot and humid and it reminded Virginia of her parents. Her mother had passed away by this time and gone on to wherever. She had been very ready to die. She used to complain that all of her friends had gone and she was the only one left. Even before her death Virginia had felt she had moved on. From time to time she felt her father's presence even though he had died years earlier. He had not wanted to die at all and maybe he was hanging around checking up on her.

When they saw some signs of life at the Institute, they went to look for the therapy room where they found a group of other people participating in the workshop. The small group chatted in the large room that contained half a dozen massage tables and a curious looking spherical contraption with a table in the middle of it located in the far corner. Three women emerged from an office and Kelly, a slim woman with long blond hair tied in a ponytail, introduced herself as lead therapist. Other therapists filtered in later. Kelly led the way into an adjoining room where they sat in a circle (on chairs this time) and introduced themselves. The other participants were also each accompanied by a support person. Eric, a boy of about eight, had been diagnosed with ADHD[222] and had his mom with him. A young woman, Janet, was suffering hallucinations as a result of an immunization regime which she had taken while traveling abroad. Her husband had come with her. Sandra was also accompanied by her husband who helped her in and out of her wheelchair. She had suffered a severe accident and was unable to walk. Lori arrived a bit late with apologies for her friend who was parking the car. She was suffering from unusual sleep disorders and bad dreams.

Moving around the circle, each participant in turn spoke briefly about the problems he or she hoped to overcome and the companion affirmed what the participant had said. The companion was also asked to describe how he or she felt and what he or she was experiencing in the situation. Virginia flashed back to that first week with Harriet when she was asked to give a purpose for being there. This time, she was ready to come up with something more. Of course, she was there to support her daughter, but it was more than that. The most important thing to Virginia was that Nicola was alive and was not going to die from another brain hemorrhage, but she could see Nicola was suffering as a result of the surgery and she would do anything to improve the situation. So, there they were: a small group of people, some of whom felt this was their last resort. The therapists concurred that many people end up in their intensive workshop after they have exhausted most other possibilities.

The morning check-in, which happened at the beginning of each day, was followed by a short meditation and then each participant went with a therapist, or maybe two, to a massage table in the large room for a craniosacral session. At that time, the companions could leave and come back at lunchtime. After lunch, there were more sessions until the end of the afternoon. A psychologist took people, in turns, into a separate room to talk. Once a week an acupuncturist came to administer his craft in conjunction with the craniosacral therapy. Sometimes, a musician came and played during a session and the spherical frame turned out to be a sound chamber which played surround sound music during a therapy session. Dr. Upledger came in one day and worked with each person individually.

At the end of the two weeks, there was an assessment of progress or change. Nicola's balance had definitely improved and she had increased sensation in her left limbs. She could also feel the floor with the bottom of her foot, something she had not been able to do since the surgery. As Virginia was continually reminded, the brain takes its time processing new information and so changes continued to occur long after their return home from the clinic. They both felt encouraged by the results and by the optimism of the clinic and the therapists. With a deep sigh, Virginia decided to continue with her therapy pursuits with the hope of no more strange encounters or visions.

Shortly after returning from the Upledger Institute with Nicola, Virginia found an office space in a nearby city. She shared the facility with other practitioners who were using different modalities, including an esthetician. She divided her time between clients who came to the office and elderly residents at care facilities and also took on a volunteer position at a cancer clinic. The clinic had a large cliental and it was unusual to see the same person twice. Since the clients were cognitively present, unlike many of those in the care facilities, Virginia could have a useful talk with them after the session and get feedback. One particular time stood out.

Virginia had never before worked with the middle-aged woman who lay on the massage table on her back, fully clothed, as was the norm for the therapy modality Virginia was using. The woman closed her eyes and heaved a deep sigh. Virginia assessed her energy and positioned herself on her client's left side. She lightly placed her hands on the woman's mid-section and the woman immediately remarked she had put one hand directly on the site of the offending tumor. Virginia did not have that information prior to the session because she found it could sometimes be distracting to know too much about the person's condition. She looked for the here and now problem, which could be completely separate from any specific diagnosis. That particular time Virginia was led to the site of the cancer. She waited for the woman's body to respond to her energy. Nothing much seemed to be happening and she felt herself move into that altered state, almost as if she was asleep but still aware of her surroundings. It was then the vivid image came to her. It was a large bowl of green lettuce, crisp and glistening from having just been washed. It was bright green, day-glow. No missing it. There was a message with the image: "Forget the lettuce; it's not important." Virginia didn't know what to make of it and, although she was starting to get used to strange visions, that was the first time there had been a voice attached. At the end of the session Virginia mentioned it to the client. *Well*, the woman said, *it's funny you say that. I really love salad and my doctor just told me a couple of days ago that I shouldn't eat it. I have been trying all kinds of things like boiling it and frying it.* Of course Virginia had no knowledge of the lettuce before the session. Virginia's impression was the woman's body was trying to tell her something and she wasn't listening. Virginia, on the other hand, was listening so the woman's subconscious told her instead.

On another occasion, a different woman was lying on the table and, during the session, Virginia picked up an image. That time it was a tall, dark-haired man, nicely dressed in a tan jacket with a tie. The message was: *He means well. He is a good man. Give him another chance.* After the session, she described the man and her client explained that was the man with whom she had just broken up. She felt he was pressuring her into marriage and she was not sure of him. When Virginia told her about the message, she thought it would help her make up her mind.[223] On both occasions, Virginia didn't know what to think. Later she discovered that she had experienced communication from the non-conscious of her client through energy. In both cases, the energy system of the other person was telling her a truth which needed to be heard in order to correct an imbalance. Energy can only tell the truth.[224] Virginia had certainly been in an altered state when the visions came to her.

Visions also came from clients at the care facilities. Here, the people were often unable to communicate in a conventional way, so she could not discuss the images with them afterward. One day, during the latter stages of Sandra's disease, when Virginia was particularly in tune with her, she sat with her eyes closed and her hands drawn to the left side of Sandra's abdomen. Suddenly a pair of pretty, pristine party shoes appeared. They were very happy shoes, floating in the sunlight. Virginia knew the memory was coming from Sandra and later spoke about it with her daughter who recounted a story from her mother's childhood. Sandra's aunt had given her a pair of new party shoes shortly before the family was to move to a rural community. On her first day at her new school, Sandra insisted on wearing her new shoes; she was so delighted with them. All the other children wore heavy boots because it was wet and muddy and the new shoes came home ruined. Sandra had often told that story in later years. On the day of Virginia's vision, she may have been remembering that time in her life and how she had loved those shoes.

From these and other experiences, Virginia noticed whenever such a vision arose she had been in that altered state. It is the state when the brain waves are in theta, which is slower than alpha but not as slow as delta (when we are asleep) or high delta (when we are dreaming).[225] Although it feels like a day-dream or a trance, she was completely aware of her surroundings, but she felt a bit fuzzy, like she was about to fall asleep at any moment. She didn't do anything special to enter this state. It just happened. She was present, in her altered state, not consciously doing much of anything other than connecting with her client, when a vision appeared. The visions were unsolicited and always clearly remembered afterward. Virginia realized her experiences, although out of the ordinary for her, must signify something. In time she recognized she had made a connection with the other person on a non-conscious level. Spontaneous imagery, such as described above, is a means of bringing the non-conscious into our conscious awareness. It occurs in a deep state of relaxation of body and mind when the controlling and logical left hemisphere of the brain relaxes its grip and the wisdom and emotion of the right hemisphere can be heard.[226]

Entering this altered state of deep relaxation can occur in different ways. Chi gong masters go to great lengths to prepare themselves to enter this altered state. It is at that time they can direct healing energy to the patient.[227] Some psychics and other healers also make elaborate preparations with candles, incense and sometimes crystals before a healing session.[228] As well as crystals, shamanic traditions use sacred pipes in ritual ceremonies to reinforce the important belief that change will take place. These *props* aid the healer, as well as the sick person, to enter an altered state where reorganization of the field can take place.[229]

Dreams are a connection to the non-conscious and can segue to changes in lifestyle, which can improve health. Sometimes, a dream can abstract the content, especially if it is related to a past trauma, and put it into another context. The dream might not make sense and might need some digging to find the real meaning.[230] A dream may also be a mind-body connection trying to express itself on a conscious level and can give guidance toward preventing a potential problem.[231] Often, dreams are health-related and appear to be a precognition of a future event.[232]

In a more purposeful manner, any practice employing focused concentration will access the mind-body connection and elicit what Herbert Benson calls the "relaxation response."[233] This is the state, opposite to high alert fight-or-flight, where the mind and body enter total relaxation.[234] It is in this state of awareness that we can access the non-conscious.[235] Benson claims there is no "Benson technique for eliciting the relaxation response."[236] Hypnosis, for example, can also provide such an entrée. Under hypnosis, a person is focusing on a single thing and able to ignore all other stimuli. In this trance-like state, one is mentally alert and able to recognize cues, but the body responds according to what the mind tells it, regardless of reality.[237] A past emotional trauma can be re-experienced, followed by a change in a present physical condition such as banishing pain.[238] Hypnosis can also be seen as a means of accessing the non-local field and thereby connecting with other individuals.[239] Guided imagery employs hypnosis to "induce a state of light trance and openness to the unconscious mind." Through a series of prompts from the therapist, the patient is encouraged to look inside at the troubling incident causing pain or illness and begin a dialogue with that part of the body. This is another form of self-awareness with the assistance of a trained therapist.[240]

Transcendental Meditation (TM) is a specific form of meditation founded by His Holiness Maharishi Mahesh Yogi.[241] It is usually practiced in a seated posture with eyes closed and incorporating the repetition of a single word. The word repetition is called a mantra. Although in practice it uses techniques of focusing the mind, the effect is a "physiologic relaxation."[242] Through TM, the mind enters a state of quiet awareness called Transcendental Consciousness. This is a state of consciousness between waking and dreaming that connects with the inner self. It is thought to be the "field of maximum energy, creativity, and intelligence."[243] Its practice has been demonstrated to have multiple physiological benefits, including reducing stress in the mind and body. It develops an increased awareness of consciousness, which translates to awareness of other individuals and relationships.[244] Although TM is considered to be a practice and not a religion or a philosophy,[245] it is derived from Eastern religions such as Hinduism and Buddhism.

Biofeedback is a Western approach which also promotes a form of self-awareness and is often used for pain management. Through the use of a computer monitor, biofeedback gives the patient visual conformation of how his or her bodily systems are behaving. It answers questions like: How does my body react physically to my thoughts and actions? Can I control the way my body reacts? As with hypnosis, the patient is asked to concentrate on a single aspect of the body. Sensors attached to the body monitor physiological occurrences like breathing, the heart rate or muscle tension. The patient gets feedback from these functions by watching the patterns on a computer screen attached to the sensors.[246] In this way, the patient is able to watch his or her biological actions and reactions and therefore learn to change heart rate or muscle tension at will. The practice increases self-awareness of the body.[247] The patient might be told, *Think a dark thought or imagine you are really mad about something and watch the screen.* As you get even more upset, you watch your heart rate, accompanied by blood pressure, rise at an alarming rate. How can you get your blood pressure back to normal?

Take a deep breath, the practitioner might say. *Concentrate on slowing down your breathing. Now, think of a calm scene like a beautiful mountain lake, shimmering in the sunlight.* As you attempt to follow directions, the lines representing your heartbeat typically begin to change, creating a smoother pattern. As you calm down, the lines on the screen return to your normal state of being. This is cool. You can change the way your body functions simply by thinking about it. The voluntary control of your breathing acts as a self-regulating system which, in turn, influences the heart rate and blood pressure.[248] Repeated practice of the control will lead to learning natural self-regulation within the entire body system.[249]

It is apparent that the breath is an important tool for body management.[250] Attention to breathing has a positive effect on the body and it is also a means of entering the relaxed state, which allows us to access the non-conscious through the mind-body connection.[251] Thich Nhat Hanh in a *Dharma Talk* says about breathing:

> "Breathing in, I am aware of my whole body. This seems to be very simple, but it is extremely important. We started to come back to the breath, and after becoming one with our in-breath, now we are becoming one with our physical body. This is returning, coming back. We wandered a lot in the past, but now we are determined to come back to ourselves. The first destination is the breath, and then it is the body, and later the feelings, the perceptions, and consciousness, knowledge."[252]

Other ways of entering altered states include spiritual practices and they also encourage attention to breath. In the Eastern traditions of Hinduism and Buddhism, meditation is common. Hatha yoga, based on Hindu tradition, has similar concepts to Chinese yin and yang. "Ha" is the positive and "tha" is the negative. Through the practice of yoga, we experience the union of the two in the central nervous system. Body postures (asanas) are assumed and they either activate or calm the central nervous system, sending information "to all the systems and organs of the body."[253] To fully experience the benefits of yoga, you must be present in the here and now in both mind and body. It is then that you can begin to listen to your mind and body speak, which has the benefit of increasing clarity in your consciousness. By using the breath in meditation, we come to a unity with mind, body and spirit and become one with God. As we move into the place of clarity, the breath becomes continuous so there is no beginning or end. This is the place of "God Consciousness" where time does not exist and we find unity with all other beings.[254] As with other disciplines, the body is impacted. Dr. Elmer Green has investigated comparisons between the physiologic effects of yoga and biofeedback.[255]

The Buddhist tradition of meditation known as mindfulness (vipassana) also uses attention to the breath and induces a calm state, reducing stress and pain.[256] Using mindfulness we notice the breath and, entering a relaxed state, we can reduce stress in the mind and also the body.[257] In Buddhist terms, it is dropping into a place of "pure mind" where there is peace and happiness.[258] Happiness is attained by training the mind to discard negative thoughts and keep the positive. Through this regular training, it is possible to reprogram the neurotransmitters in the brain and achieve a new and healthier state of happiness.[259] Meditation can lead into the state of being present in body and mind. Both hypnosis and mediation use tools of focusing on something, or nothing, to access the non-conscious state.[260] In this state, a person can choose to use his own non-conscious levels to understand or even influence what is going on in the body.[261] This is the state where you are more likely to be able to accept visions coming from a connection with someone else.

Prayer uses concentration similar to meditation. Reciting a liturgy has a rhythmical, repetitive sound and some Christian and Eastern religions include beads, such as the rosary in the Catholic tradition, which have a repetitive motion helping the mind to focus.[262] Any ritual can have the same effect. This is particularly significant when it comes to praying for someone who is ill or in need. The energy that originates with God "energizes the whole system of Nature."[263]   In

Christian traditions, prayer allows us to enter the energetic layer of the universe and communicate with the sick person. The result has been described as a feeling of bonding with the object of intention.[264] The energy of Nature, which originates with God, gives the body healing assistance.[265] St. Teresa of Avila writes on mystical theology and in the writings of her Life, she records visions and messages from God.[266] Healing can also occur when the recipient of prayer is not present. It is now called distance healing. Examples in the Bible include the healing of the centurion's servant by Jesus.[267] Other forms of Christian faith such as Christian Science, Pentecostalism, Scientology, Spiritualism, etc. employ various methods to promote healing and communication with God.[268]

All of these practices involving the mind enable you to access another level of your being, a level outside the normal conscious one. It is on this level that the mind and energy operate and it is also here that we are able to communicate with each other in ways not normally thought of as traditional. In the arena of quantum energy, the healing prayers or good wishes enter the field and are transmitted to the recipient. Whether it is thought of in terms of benevolent intervention by God or a Creator, in terms of healing energy in the field, or in terms of positive chi, studies have shown faith healing or distance healing to have had positive effects on the sick.[269]

Some medical practitioners are aware non-conscious communication is possible. When Virginia's dying father went into a coma, the doctor drew her mother and herself out of the room to talk to them about his prognosis, which was not good. The doctor may have thought that there was a possibility her father could hear and understand the conversation even though he was technically unconscious. Patients under anesthetic during surgery have awakened to repeat the conversations that took place while they were out.[270] A recent article in the New York Times reported a study of a "brain-damaged woman in an unresponsive, vegetative state [who] showed clear signs on brain imaging tests that she was aware of herself and her surroundings. . ."[271] Although doctors know this can happen, most are reluctant to discuss it because bio-medical science has not yet fully explained it. Perhaps the most recent findings will be a cornerstone for new communication.

It is not necessary to have psychic powers to experience this type of communication. Reading energy fields is a skill that can be acquired.[272] Virginia certainly knew that she did not have any special gifts. Anyone can do this; all that is necessary is to be open and available to the opportunity. A therapist who is trained in this type of work will be able to communicate with a client in this manner. Even better, a family member who already knows the person well can easily tap into the non-conscious. The family member may even recognize images or messages. An Alzheimer's patient who has lost the power of speech can still convey images. It is important to remember not everyone feels chatty all the time. People who do talk constantly can be kind of annoying. The person with whom you are trying to connect may not feel like talking at that moment. Don't give up and think it won't happen. Keep at it. Communication may not come in the form of a vision, as described above. It may be a feeling or an awareness that the person knows you are there and you will feel a sense of connection and completeness. It may even be healing for you as well as your loved one.

Chapter 9

The Healers

Early on in this work, when Virginia was still trying to figure out what she was doing, she found very little information or real support. She came across a course entitled "Working with the Elderly and Terminally Ill" at McKinnon Institute of Massage in Oakland, CA. This course appealed to her immediately because, at last, she had found others who were experiencing the same challenges. Nowhere else had she seen a class devoted to her population.[273] Virginia hoped to get some clues about things she was doing wrong, could do better or differently, or new approaches that might give different results. She hoped to find some validation for what she had been doing, which is exactly what happened. The techniques she had adapted for her senior population were considered by others to be appropriate. Frail bodies need a light gentle touch and patience forcing her to slow down and wait for them to respond. Sometimes, the response was hard to recognize because they tended to have low energy and it could be hard to find.

A couple of people that Virginia met in the class had experience working with Hospice. Hospice is designed to offer palliative care for the terminally ill and dying. "The focus of Hospice is to ensure the comfort of every patient during the final stages of life."[274] The organization has been working hard to dispel the myth that they only help patients who are suffering from cancer and are expected to die within six months. The services are intended for those suffering from *life-limiting* illness and for some patients this may be a year or longer.[275] A patient must however have a *good-faith prognosis* of six months or less to live in order to be accepted in the first place. "The six-month diagnosis is fixed by the Hospice Medicare Benefits, and followed by most private insurance companies."[276] Services offered include nursing, physician care, pharmacy, home health aide, and social services. In addition, Hospice offers support for family members and valuable grief counseling following a death. There is also a network of volunteers who are assigned a patient to visit. They cover a range of routine tasks such as errand running and light housework but some also provide hair dressing and massage therapy.

With a disease such as Alzheimer's, the progression is slow and may continue over many years. It is improbable that a prediction can be made as to the length of life remaining. Although Hospice offers services for Alzheimer's patients, it is unclear when their involvement may start due to the difficult nature of the disease. Other brain related diseases have the same problem. So it was with Virginia's mother who was suffering from dementia but was otherwise not unwell. Hospice would not take her as a client because there was no projected time of death. Her father was given only a short time to live and when her mother brought Hospice in, he was distressed at the idea because he considered their involvement to be a death sentence. He felt that everyone had given up on him. Hospice says that this is not an uncommon reaction. They say emphatically that their focus is "comfort, quality of life and support 24 hours a day."[277] Many people do have good experiences with Hospice and they do provide a valuable service relieving family and caregivers from some of the strain of dealing with death. The organization is blessed with compassionate volunteers. The intention is to offer support and comfort, not to heal. Sometimes touch is incorporated, sometimes not. Holding the patient's hands is encouraged[278] but connection to the non-conscious levels appears to be out of the scope for the volunteers. Spiritual counselors come closest to this and are most helpful during the last stages of life.

Talk of healing tends to be in terms of illness in the physical body, but the other levels making up the individual can suffer from injury or illness as well, and they could also be in need of healing. Sometimes, it is illness on the other levels that eventually manifests as physical illness. All levels need to be addressed in order to bring about good health to the whole person. Virginia never thought of herself as a healer. In fact, she was quite sure she did not have any special powers to heal anyone. Some people profess to have such abilities and indeed, they may. Practitioners of intuitive healing are able to sense, through their intuition, the nature and location of an illness. Using the person's energy, they can locate a tumor or diagnose kidney failure. They assist the patient to call on their own inner strength and spirit to effect a change in the physical, mental or spiritual body. They are positive in attitude and it seems to work, although they generally work in cooperation with a biomedical doctor, not in place of one.

It is the positive that must be emphasized. "Beware of negative messages," says Dr. Judith Orloff. "Insensitive healers are notorious for toxic pronouncements."[279] How often did Virginia sit in a physical therapy gym with her daughter, only to be insensitively told by the therapist that her child would not have any further improvement. Dr. Orloff calls this type of pronouncement not only "just irresponsible" but says that it "can do real harm."[280] Nicola would invariably be very upset after such an incident and rush out crying. It took some time to calm her down and convince her that they both believed she would improve.

Sometimes, intuitive healers use a hands-on approach, sometimes it is remote. As in chi gong and Pranic Healing, it is possible to affect the energy without touching the person. Intuitive healers do this. The energy field extends beyond the physical body, so working off the body can be effective. Pranic

Healing uses a sweeping, cleansing motion with the hands to clear blockages or to move universal energy into holes in the person's field. It is also possible to promote healing without the motions by using intention. This form of off-the-body healing is done in the immediate aura or energy field of the sick person. It follows that through the universal field, or zero point field, healing could be effective at a great distance. Sometimes called distance healing, there are similarities with prayer healing which can be very powerful. Although no one is sure exactly how it works and there are theories including non-locality, controlled studies have shown "statistically significant results" that distance healing has occurred.[281] Some of those studied were shown to be able to influence their own bodies through healing thoughts and, when large groups were studied, healing results were consistent, regardless of the target. Whether it was through prayer or healing thoughts directed toward another at a distance, healing did occur for that person.[282]

There are occasions when a doctor may invite such a healer into the operating room during surgery.[283] The healer connects with the non-conscious level of the patient and helps guide the patient through the operation. It may be hard to tell if the results would have been different if the healer hadn't been there. Some healers suggest calling on inner guidance, which may appear in the form of an angel, a wise ancestor, an animal or whatever comes into your awareness. You can find your guide through prayer, meditation or any other way that leads into your non-conscious subtle energy. This is another way of asking your inner self for assistance with a problem.[284] Healing guides can help point the way toward whatever you might be overlooking in terms of healing.[285] It can be physical, psychological, spiritual or emotional healing that is needed. Your guide will know. It may be the health of someone else that is in question. Your guide can help there, too. All you have to do is ask. Anyone who takes the time to learn about it can elicit similar responses.

Shamans and native healers also connect with the non-conscious part of the patient.[286]   In tribal settings, the shaman is the wise one who can guide the sick person toward the healing "knowledge" which lies in his non-conscious.[287]   He or she acts as an instrument of the Creator and is, therefore, knowing and powerful. Using traditional tribal ceremonies, the shaman can call on the spirit and energy of the sick person, believing emotional and physical healing will follow.[288] Spirits will also promote visions to help guide the sick person toward a resolution.[289] The work with a shaman is intense and usually focused into a short time frame.[290]

There is some discussion about healing through channeled energy, also called psychokinesis (PK), which produces a healing force, as opposed to the body's own amazing capacity to self-heal, induced by psychological or physical placebos.[291] PK may actually be an integration of universal and vital energies because the self, in its awareness, will feel the presence of the healing force and act accordingly. Although channeling has some similarities to nineteenth century Spiritualism,[292] it is thought to be New Age. Channels invoke spiritual guides to help resolve conflicts, which may have come from an earlier life and are now manifesting as an illness.[293]

Biomedicine, herbs and other remedies help our bodies fend off disease and ease pain. However, according to David Shenk in what he calls "the art of living – and dying," medicine alone cannot show us the way to healing.[294] Human connection, on the other hand, is helpful. Non-pharmacologic therapies, such as gentle massage, have been shown to relieve pain in the elderly and terminally ill. They can be successfully used in conjunction with conventional drug-based pain management.[295]

The real healing is, however, done by the sick person. Sometimes, it seems as though the body and mind are not aware there is a problem. The person is distracted and it goes unnoticed. A therapist might be able to bring attention to the problem so the body can do its work. This self-healing can be instigated by a therapist, in collaboration with the client, through intention, manipulation of energy, or suggestion. There are many hands-on techniques, as well as non-touch techniques, which offer this type of assistance. Whatever the technique, the outcome points to the amazing ability of the body to heal itself.[296] It is important to realize non-conventional therapies and healing modalities should not take the place of biomedicine but be used in conjunction with it. If you were hit by a bus, you would want to go the emergency room, not be given herbal tea or have your aura cleansed.

Many different therapies are offered, some in the bio-medical realm and some in the complimentary/alternative arena. Ultimately, it seems to be a matter for the individual to find the therapy – it could be an accumulation of therapies - which creates their healing, that moment when internal change can make healing possible.[297] All modalities can create healing. It's like trying them on for size. Whatever avenue you choose, the results will depend on your presence and participation.

It is difficult to imagine someone in the later stages of Alzheimer's disease, whose conventional communication is dysfunctional, being able to cognitively affect his or her own healing or a change in his or her health status. For elderly and frail people or those suffering from brain disorders such as stroke or the various dementias, it may not be possible for the body to effect physical healing. The word "healing" can be misleading. With the Alzheimer's patient, the healing needed could be on a level other than the physical. Physiological healing might be improbable, if not impossible, but what may be of greatest help to the person is emotional or spiritual healing, or a sense of complete self or wholeness. It could mean finishing something left unsaid or undone. Physical healing sometimes follows.[298] It is most important to acknowledge that, whatever changes may occur, physical healing may or may not be a part of it. Virginia realized when she touched her clients they felt less abandoned, more valued and wanted, less likely to give up and they might try to get better. The intention is simply to communicate and to offer a helping hand and a non-judgmental space for healing to occur. A connection with the person on a non-conscious level will help the person to discern the real healing need.

Once you understand the connection, you can tell if something is bothering your loved one. You can reassure them that those things are taken care of and they don't have to worry about it any more. Getting that message across can be a great help. Virginia's mother was fed up, uncomfortable and didn't want to live anymore. She hung on until she was satisfied Virginia and her family would be all right. Sometimes, people feel guilty about dying. Virginia's father felt he was letting her mother down and that he had a lot more to do in this life. Virginia didn't know what to do at the time, but later she realized she could have given reassurance that she loved him, was there for him, and she was not giving up on him. With her daughter she refused to listen to anyone say that she might die because she *knew* Nicola would be all right. The difference with her father was in their relationship. He was the parent and, although he was sick, she felt he was in charge. That may have been why she had such a hard time with her mother who was always in the parent role and yet Virginia found herself having to take charge and unfamiliar with this role reversal.

Virginia's clients who were not suffering from Alzheimer's or other forms of dementia sometimes expected a more conventional massage approach. Nevertheless, they were also frail and had little muscle mass and they still required a special light treatment. In fact, Virginia noticed very light pressure felt intense to them. She did not intend to move the tissue around too much; she used the same light touch, waiting for the body to respond. Their bodies were compromised in some way and it was important to honor their years of use and misuse. There was also wisdom in those bodies and much can be learned from them.

Victoria was a fastidious lady who loved her jewelry and liked to have her hair and make up just so. She was in constant pain, however, and the family thought some massage might give her some relief. Just touching her caused discomfort, but she liked to have her feet rubbed. Through foot reflexology,[299] Virginia could work on her entire body and she did receive some benefit from this technique.

Another resident, Lucy, reminded Virginia a lot of her mother. Some time after she moved to the care facility, Virginia was contacted by the facility because the family had requested massage. Lucy had tension in her neck and shoulders and the family thought some massage would help. When Virginia found her room, she introduced herself and knelt by the side of her bed. Virginia gently took her hand and asked how she was feeling. As expected, she was non-committal. She asked Lucy's permission to stroke her head. She loved it. Each time she remarked how good it felt. Lucy also loved having her feet rubbed. Virginia used light pressure, slowly and gently moving across her socks. Working on Lucy's left side, her affected side, was as necessary as on her right side and it needed an equal amount of attention. Her left arm was sometimes stiff, but after working with it for a few minutes it loosened up. All of this took about a half hour. Virginia started seeing her once a week. After a few visits, Lucy said she could have an hour massage. Virginia's reply was always that an hour is too long. When the person's system is severely compromised, the body will only respond for a short period. Lucy and Virginia solved the problem by having a half hour massage twice a week. She often said Virginia could stay all day.

During the course of her sessions with Lucy, Virginia discovered how she came to be in the care facility and how she felt about it. Lucy and her husband had been married for forty-seven years when suddenly, he died. Lucy was so distraught by the loss of her partner that she, in turn, suffered a stroke. *Well, now what?* Lucy thought. Her whole left side was paralyzed and she obviously couldn't care for herself in

that condition. She didn't want to be a burden. How long
before she would be better? Ted, her only child, lived miles
away. He and his wife, Susan, showed up at the hospital.
Susan bustled around the hospital room while Ted stood over
the bed. *Mom, we are going to move you closer to us,* he told
her. What exactly does that mean? It meant, as she found out,
a "skilled nursing facility" or a nursing home. What about her
own home? Ted was arranging to sell it and move the contents
to his home or into storage. Didn't she have any say in the
matter? Well, no. Susan said it was for the best. Then they
could visit her often.

It seemed like a nice enough place. Lucy had a
roommate who called out from time to time. At least, she
had a TV of her own. She could watch TV all day, especially
the chat shows. The trouble that people get into! She and
her husband never had problems like that; Ted was a model
child, never any trouble. How long would she be here? She
was looking forward to having her own place again. She
missed cooking and she wondered where all her household
possessions were. Would she ever see them again? She missed
her husband terribly. Thinking of him made her cry. Was she
going to die here? She had a dull life really, or so she had told
Virginia. Oh, Dr. Phil is on . . . Lucy was easily distracted.

During the sessions with Lucy, they talked about
whatever was on her mind at the time. Sometimes, Virginia
would come in and find her in tears, thinking about her
husband, and they would talk about past times with him. Other
times, the conversation would steer toward the future for her
or events in the news. Lucy did not suffer from dementia,
her hearing was good and, when her glasses were not broken,
she could see a bit. Her only real problem was the lack of
control of her left side, a result of the stroke. This alone had
landed her in a nursing home. Not all of Virginia's clients
are as straight forward as Lucy. The people suffering from
Alzheimer's disease and other forms of dementia clearly
present different problems.

When an Alzheimer's patient is past the knowing-that-something-is-wrong stage, which at best or at worst is infrequent, their feelings about life are on the non-conscious level. That does not make it any less painful or frustrating for them than if they were conscious of what is going on. Appropriate gentle touch can certainly benefit the elderly, those with chronic pain and those with dementia.[300] Slow stroke massage by caregivers has been shown to decrease agitation in Alzheimer's patients,[301] and it could come from hospital or nursing home staff, but problems exist. Lack of massage training, lack of time and general indifference gets in the way. [302] Caregivers and nursing aids could improve their level of communication with nursing home residents[303] but unfortunately, such attempts seem to be short-lived.[304] Efforts are made to make the atmosphere friendly with joking interaction between staff members, but the lightheartedness is superficial, in an attempt to relieve what can be a difficult and depressing environment. As nursing homes have notorious staffing problems, this situation has little hope of changing. That leaves it up to family members or another designated person to fill in the support and connection gap.

Many of the seniors in care facilities with whom Virginia has worked have huge barriers and also have depleted vital energy or chi. When healing, or comfort, is needed, the barriers make it hard to discover the source for concern. She met Roger's wife, Sally, one day at the care facility. Roger's Alzheimer's was advanced. His movements were uncontrolled and he was unable to speak. He slept most of the time and when he was awake, he had a vacant stare. Sally said he would enjoy some massage, so Virginia began working with him. Roger had a military background and had been the family provider, responsible for everything, especially Sally. He could not let go of that. It took many months to connect with Roger. He sat in the dining room strapped into his wheelchair, his neck and shoulders like boulders. His energy was low and very guarded. He tried hard to ignore Virginia, but it took a lot of effort. He would fall asleep, but he was still tense. Virginia kept at it, repeating the same motions resting her hands on his shoulders and waiting. Finally, there was a glimmer of connection. It was difficult to read. He began to relax when she touched him and she was able to reassure him that Sally was being taken care of and he didn't have to worry about her. Roger didn't believe her and continued his stare. It was tough.

Sometimes Virginia's clients were perfectly content with life and happy to just hang out. She had been visiting Joan regularly for about seven years. At first, she would find her in her wheelchair and she would chew on her fingers and repeatedly count, *six, seven, eight . . . six, seven, eight.* From the stories her husband had told Virginia, she was an intelligent and accomplished professional woman. Her energy had always been strong, but it also had a locked–up quality. It was hard for Virginia to get through to her. Her body was tense and she fidgeted. After a few years she stopped counting, or saying anything, but she did become calmer. One day, Virginia had a vision from her, a colorful stocking cap. *Where did that come from?* she wondered. She asked Joan's husband about it and he immediately replied, *I know that hat. She always wore it to games. She was a huge Raiders' fan.* At last, she was talking. It had taken years, but Virginia noticed a little giving to her touch. In Joan's case, Virginia's presence seemed to reassure her that someone was there. There was a constant and things could go on.

Doris loved to garden. She liked nothing better than going outside on the patio and digging around in the dirt. The activities staff would bring in small potted plants for her to put in the garden. She had a great time muttering away about the garden; sometimes her words made sense, sometimes not. Although Doris recognized the garden and the plants, she didn't do quite so well with people. When Virginia arrived Doris never remembered her but as Virginia placed her hand on Doris' shoulder, she always answered positively right away and as her back and shoulders were massaged, she would make soft purring noises.

Ultimately, we each have to find our own way in life and getting lost seems to be part of the journey. Especially when one becomes infirm, or is suffering, support and reassurance is helpful. No one can tell another person which path to choose or how to travel it. What one can do is witness their journey and accept the chosen way. This is the most powerful reassurance we can offer. Simply being present and staying by the person's side is a tremendous boost. He or she is being seen. Whatever their decision, it is accepted without judgment. Although distance support and connection through the field is powerful, touching another human being is the easiest and most direct way to offer this kind of support.

Much of this discussion has revolved around people suffering from Alzheimer's disease. It has been discussed in depth, partly because of experience, but also because of the longevity and extent of care required. The lessons from the Alzheimer's sufferers apply to anyone in a care situation and anyone suffering. The need for communication, support and witness is equal. If your grandma is cognitively present, you can visit her and stop by on a regular basis just to say *hi*. A brief visit is all that is necessary. A person in a situation when, due to age or illness, they are unable to move in normal social circles and relate to others will find it helpful if a family member or a designated other can visit regularly and provide support. It is clear this is helpful in the psychological arena.[305] If you are having a bad day, the fact that someone notices can make you feel better. Touch enhances and reinforces this connection and gives reassurance that the person is not alone. For the dementia patient, it is the same. They are still present on the non-conscious level and appreciate that you stop by. You don't have to stay long. When you touch them, they know it's you. It makes all the difference. The connection encourages changes and healing on whatever level, and you are the healer.

Although energy is present in all living things, it is not necessary to use energy therapy, or even to understand it or believe in it, in order to work with seniors. The energies of the two people will interact naturally. Neither person has to do anything other than show up. For the trained therapist, energy can be a powerful tool. It can be restored and directed to aid the body in healing, whatever kind of healing is needed. As people age or if they suffer from an illness, their energy tends to get weaker and more difficult to track. Touch with presence and compassion will have the effect of saying: *I am here; I see what you are going through; you are not alone.*[306] It is not offering to change it or fix it but is offering a non-judgmental caring presence.[307]

Chapter 10

Cactus

There is some indication that the focus of long-term care facilities will change in the near future. With the soon to be increasing senior population, the boomers, there is discussion that the model will become less medically oriented and more focused on the care recipients themselves, their desires and needs. Whether or not this change includes technological advances in the care-giving realm, which seems to be an increasing possibility, hopefully the real shift will be toward recognizing the individual in need of long-term care, whether at home or in an institution, is still a person who hasn't disappeared and his or her preferences should be honored. Striving to retain communication, verbal or not, must be a priority. Touch is such a simple and effective means of sustaining a connection. Replacing the personal visit by a telephone call, although better than nothing, is hardly as satisfactory.

As far as connecting with your loved one, those who have a strong faith in God, or a higher power, may have an advantage. It is their very belief that will carry them through to the non-conscious connection. They believe God will help them and so He will. They are open to the possibility. Those who are not so passionate about religion may need to look for other avenues such as meditation. For them also, it is necessary to be open to the idea. Whatever avenue you choose, it is the attitude and willingness to connect or be with your loved one that makes the difference.[309] Your loved one will benefit and so will you.

When someone mentions cactus, the first thing Virginia thinks of is sharp or prickly spikes. It is not something she would want to pick up and stroke or hold lovingly in her hands. Cacti come in all sizes and shapes. Some of them are round and bulbous and some have angular appendages. They are prickly and spiky but they are soft inside and they also have beautiful blooms. Spectacular, even! Some years ago, a friend gave her a cactus as a thank-you gift. It was a sizable plant with several hand-like appendages growing out and up from a short squat center. Virginia was a little mystified and stuck it in a corner on the deck. There it sat for ten years, being ignored. It didn't grow; it didn't bloom; it didn't die. It just sat there. It looked pretty ugly. It turned out her friend had raised this cactus from birth and he was very proud of it. It undoubtedly deserved better treatment than it had received. Perhaps it does have great potential, even though it has been sitting there for years. Its variety, she had been told, can have beautiful blooms. Sadly, the beauty of her cactus was masked by neglect.

By now, you can see the parallel with seniors. They also come in all sizes and shapes and with different backgrounds and stories. Some are angry and resentful; some are quiet and accepting; some are in another dimension. Leave them to sit in their wheelchairs and they will do just that – sit. But a quiet, gentle and persistent presence can bring out the bloom. They all have stories. They love to tell them. Sometimes they can verbalize them and sometimes not. It is always possible to listen even if it is not verbal. Being persistent and regular is key. It doesn't have to be long, just regular. The bloom is always beautiful and worth the wait. Remember, we will all be there some day.

Virginia has moved her cactus into the kitchen next to an orchid that is about to bloom. Maybe it will take the hint. She talks to it regularly now. Last week, she was very excited to notice a new little arm growing from the side of her cactus. This is the first time in all these years there has been any new growth or signs of life. It has always looked crusty and lifeless on the outside. For a while, Virginia actually thought it was dead. Just yesterday, she was inspecting it and trying to clean off some of the more unsightly bits. One of the arms fell right off. Perhaps that bit was dead but underneath she found a second new bit of growth. It is very much alive inside and now growing again; even getting a little carried away. Hurray!

Endnotes

1   *Geriatric Review Syllabus 5th* ed. (New York: American
    Geriatrics Society, 2004), 8.

2   *The State of Aging and Health in America* (Merck Institute of
    Aging & Health, The Gerontological Society of America,
    2003). Available from http://www.agingsociety.org/
    agingsociety/pdf/state_of_aging_report.pdf.
    (accessed May, 2006).

3   *Facts on Long Term Care* (Washington DC: National Academy
    on Aging, September, 1997).

4   *The State of Aging and Health in America.*

5   *Facts on Long Term Care.*

6   American Association of Homes and Services for the Aging
    (April 2, 2006). Available from http://www.2.aahsa.org.
    (accessed May, 2006)

7   *Public Policy & Aging Report* (Washington, D.C.: National
    Academy on an Aging Society and The Gerontological Society
    of America 15(4), Fall 2005).

8   Robyn I. Stone, *Long-Term Care of the Elderly with Disabilities*
    (New York: Milbank Memorial Fund, August, 2000).

9   Judith Viorst, *Necessary Losses* (New York: The Free Press,
    1986), 223.

10 Julia Huber, *The New Old – How Baby Boomers are Redefining
    Retirement* (AARP Policy & Research, July, 2004). Available
    from http://www.aarp.org/research/reference/boomers/a2004-
    07-22-globalperspectives.html. (accessed April, 2006).

11 Larry Dossey, M.D., *Healing Beyond the Body* (Boston:
    Shambhala Publications Inc., 2001), 136-139.

12   Michelle Weinstein, *Laughter is the 'Best Medicine' for Your Heart* (University of Maryland Medical Center). Available from http://www.umm.edu/features/laughter.htm. (accessed May, 2006).

13   *Communities for All Ages Gather Youth and Seniors from across Arizona* (Arizona Community Foundation, March 24, 2004). Available from http://www.acf.org. (accessed June, 2006).

14   Lawrence K. Grossman, "The Media's Role," *Life in an Older America* (New York: The Century Foundation Press, 1999), 213.

15   Viorst, 223.

16   *The Secret Life of the Brain.* Available from http://www.pbs.org/brain. (accessed July, 2006).

17   Sara E. Rix, "The Older Worker in a Graying America," *Life in an Older America* (New York: The Century Foundation Press, 1999), 203.

18   Viorst, 291.

19   *What Are the Attitudes of Young Retirees and Older Workers?* (Washington, D.C.: National Academy on Aging, Number 5, February, 2001). Available from http://www.agingsociety.org/agingsociety/pdf/aarp5.pdf. (accessed May, 2006).

20   Jean Carper, *Your Miracle Brain* (New York: HarperCollins, 2000), 16.

21   *Who Are Young Retirees and Older Workers?* (Washington, D.C.: National Academy on Aging, 1, June, 2000). Available from http://www. agingsociety.org/agingsociety/pdf/aarp1.pdf. (accessed May, 2006).

22   Ibid.

23   Stone, 50.

24   Neil Charness, *Age, Technology, and Culture: Gerontopia or Dystopia* (Washington D.C.: National Academy on an Aging Society and The Gerontological Society of America 15(4), Fall, 2005).

25   University of Iowa, Student Health. Available from http://www.uiowa.edu/~shs/stree2/htm.

26   Anne Fadiman, *The Spirit Catches You and You Fall Down* (New York: Farrar, Straus and Giroux, 1997), 182-183. "During the late 1910s and early '20s, immigrant workers at the Ford automotive plant in Dearborn, Michigan, were given free,

compulsory 'Americanization' classes.... During their graduation ceremony they gathered next to a gigantic wooden pot, which their teachers stirred with ten-foot ladles. The students walked through a door into the pot, wearing traditional costumes from their countries of origin and singing songs in their native languages. A few minutes later, the door in the pot opened, and the students walked out again, wearing suits and ties, waving American flags and singing 'The Star-Spangled Banner.'"

27   The altitude at Cusco is 11,156ft. See http://www.peru.info. (accessed July, 2006).

28   Seventh highest mountain in Nepal, Annapurna stands at a mere 26,545ft compared to Mt Everest at 29,028ft. See http://www. nepalhomepage.com. (accessed July, 2006).

29   Linda Tuhiwai Smith, *Decolonizing Methodologies* (New York: Zed Books, Ltd., 1999), 97.

30   Marlo Morgan, *Mutant Message Down Under* (New York: HarperCollins, 1991), 95-96.

31   Smith, 99.

32   Lori Arviso Alvord, M.D. and Elizabeth Cohen Van Pelt, *The Scalpel and the Silver Bear* (New York: Bantam Books, 2000), 113.

33   Alvord, 85.

34   Lewis Mehl-Madrona, M.D., *Coyote Medicine* (New York: Fireside, 1997), 123-126.

35   Ibid., 164.

36   Ibid., 231.

37   Alvord, 100.

38   Interview with Natasha Boissier, LCSW, Resource Center for Caregivers, "American Society on Aging, Autumn Series" (September 26, 2006), San Francisco, California.

39   Ibid.

40   Interview with Owen Lum, M.D., Indian Health Center of Santa Clara Valley, "American Society on Aging, Autumn Series" (September 26, 2006), San Francisco, California.

41   Ibid., Natasha Boissier.

42   Ibid., Owen Lum, MD.

43   *Public Policy & Aging Report.*

44   Laura Carstensen et al., *Practical Handbook of Clinical Gerontology,* (Thousand Oaks, CA: Sage Publications, Inc., 1996), 60.

45   *Normal Reactions to Loss* (AARP). Available from http://www. aarp.org/families/grief_loss/a2004-11-15-reactions.html. (accessed June, 2006).

46   Viorst, 239.

47   *Geriatric Review Syllabus* 5th ed., 18.

48   Viorst, 257.

49   *Nurse's Notes for Healthy Aging* (The Merck Institute of Aging & Health). Available from http://www.miahonline.org/ resources/nursenotes/articles/01_10_05.grief_reactions.html. (accessed July, 2006).

50   *Geriatric Review Syllabus* 5th ed., 15.

51   Ibid., 258.

52   *Nurse's Notes for Healthy Aging.*

53   Carstensen, 60-61.

54   Wendy L.Watson, *Aging is a Family Affair* (Brigham Young University, Family Studies Center). Available from http:// familycenter.byu.edu/columns.aspx?id=47. (accessed June, 2006).

55   Viorst, 270.

56   Suzanne R. Kunkel and Ian M. Nelson, *Consumer Direction: Changing the Landscape of Long-TermCare, Public Policy & Aging Report* (Washington D.C.: National Academy on an Aging Society and The Gerontological Society of America 15(4), Fall 2005).

57   Philip Slater, *Pursuit of Loneliness* (Boston: Beacon Press, 1976), 61.

58   See http://www.heirloomstories.com/seniorhealth.htm. (accessed March, 2006).

59   American Society on Aging. Available from http://www. asaging.com. (accessed May, 2006).

60   Ibid. 122.

61   Ibid.

62   *Nurse's Notes for Healthy Aging.*

63   *Facts on Long-Term Care.*

64 *Older Americans 2004: Key Indicators of Well-Being* (Federal Interagency Forum on Aging-Related Statistics). Available from http://www.agingstats.gov/chartbook2004/healthstatus.html. (accessed June, 2006).

65 *Facts on Long-Term Care.*

66 David Shenk, *The Forgetting* (New York: Anchor Books, 2003), 66.

67 Quality of Life Research Unit, Center for Function and Well-Being, University of Toronto. Available from http://www.utoronto.ca/qol/seniors.htm. (accessed August, 2006).

68 *Facts on Long Term Care.*

69 Comfort Keepers, Dayton, Ohio. Available from http://www.comfortkeepers.com. (accessed August, 2006).

70 Ivo Abraham, *Geriatric Nursing Protocols for Best Practice* (New York: Springer Publishing, 1999), 31- 46.

71 Slater, 19.

72 *Geriatric Review Syllabus* 5th ed., 10.

73 American Society on Aging. Available from http://www.asaging.com. (accessed May, 2006).

74 Charlene Harrington, Ph.D., James H. Swan, Ph.D., John A. Nyman, Ph.D., and Helen Carrillo, MS, "The Effect of Certificate of Need and Moratoria Policy on Change in Nursing Home Beds in the United States," *Medical Care* 35:6 (June 1997), 574-588.

75 Barbara Caldwell, "Certificate of Need Regulation in the Nursing Home Industry: Has It Outlived Its Usefulness?" *American Society of Health Economists* (June 2006). Available from http://healtheconomics.us/conference/2006/abstracts/topics-in-health-care-organizations/certificate_of_need_regulation_in_the_nursing_home_industry_has_it_oulived/ (accessed June, 2006).

76 "Old and Getting Older" (1999). Available from http://www.efmoody.com/longtem/aging.html (accessed May, 2006).

77 Omnibus Budget Reconciliation Act of 1987 (also known as the Nursing Home Reform Act). Consult the Nursing Home Abuse and Neglect Resource Center for a list of regulations and your rights. Available from http://www.nursinghomealert.com. (accessed July, 2006).

78 See http://www.asaging.com. (accessed May, 2006).

79 See http://www.HealthGrades.com. (accessed July, 2006).

80 Philip B. Stafford, *Creating Lifespan Communities, Public Policy and Aging Report* (Washington, D.C.: National Academy on an Aging Society and The Gerontological Society of America 15(4), Fall, 2005).

81 *Geriatrics Review Syllabus* 5th ed., 17.

82 Ibid., 122.

83 Carstensen, 4.

84 Thomas Hanna, *Somatics: Reawakening the Mind's Control of Movement, Flexibility, and Health* (Reading, Massachusetts: Perseus Books, 1988), 70.

85 Carstensen, 10.

86 Hanna, 40-41.

87 Carstensen, 12.

88 REM sleep refers to a sleep state called "rapid eye movement" when the brain is very active. It is thought that people over the age of seventy spend less than 10% of their sleep time in REM, while a newborn spends 80%. Average is 20%. See http://en.wikipedia.org/wiki/REM_sleep. (accessed September, 2006).

89 Ibid., 17.

90 Judith Orloff, M.D., *Intuitive Healing* (New York: Times Books, 2000), 75.

91 See http://www.esalen.org. (accessed June, 2006).

92 See http://wwwaagt.org. (accessed October, 2006).

93 See http:www.hannasomatics.com or http://www.somaticsed.com. (accessed October, 2006).

94 See http://www.feldenkrais-method.org. (accessed April, 2006).

95 Interview with Harriet Goslins (June 7, 2006), Laguna Beach, California.

96 See http://www.upledger.com. (accessed May, 2006).

97 John Upledger, DOM, *Your Inner Physician and You* (Berkeley, California: North Atlantic Press, 1997).

98 See http://www.nhi.edu. (accessed May, 2006).

99 See http://www.inawareness.com. (accessed June, 2006).

100 Choa Kok Sui, *Pranic Healing* (York Beach, Maine: Samuel Weiser, Inc., 1990).

101 Linda S. Noelker, "Training Direct Care Workers for Person-Centered Care," *Public Policy & Aging Report*.

102 In the State of California, Certified Nurse Assistants (CNA) must be certified by the state and are required to obtain a minimum of forty-eight hours of continuing education during the two years of certification. See http://www.dhs.ca.gov/Inc/download/cert/CNA-FAQ.pdf. (accessed August, 2006).

103 Claudia J. Strauss, *Talking to Alzheimer's* (Oakland, CA.: New Harbinger Publications, Inc., 2001), 51-52.

104 Lisa Radin and Gary Radin, eds., *What If It's Not Alzheimer's?* (New York: Prometheus Books, 2003), 29-38.

105 Shenk, 12-25.

106 *The Life and Death of a Neuron* (Bethesda, MD: National Institute of Neurological Disorders and Stroke), NIH Publication No. 02-3440d, December 8, 2005.

107 *Memory, Learning, and Emotion: the Hippocampus.* Available from http://www.psycheducation.org/emotion/hippocampus.htm. (accessed July, 2006).

108 Carper, 23.

109 National Institute on Aging, National Institutes of Health, Public Health Service, U.S. Department of Health and Human Services, April 25, 2006. Available from http://www.nia.nih.gov/Alzheimers/Publications/adfact.htm#Contents. (accessed May, 2006).

110 Carper, 292-294. Huperzine A, a drug originating in China, has outperformed donepezil and tacrine "in reversing memory deficits in aging animals." It has promise for treating Alzheimer's patients.

111 *Secret Life of the Brain.*

111 *The Life and Death of a Neuron.*

112 Novella J. Ruffin, Ph.D., *Understanding Growth and Development Patterns of Infants* (Blacksburg, VA: Virginia Polytechnic Institute and State University, June 2001), Publication Number 350-055.

113 Russell D. Hammer, Ph.D., "What Can My Baby See?" The Smith-Kettlewell Eye Research Institute, originally published in *Parents' Press*, XI(II) (November, 19 90).

114 *The Secret Life of the Brain.*

115 Shenk, 124-125.

116 Ibid., 52.

117 *The Secret Life of the Brain.*

118   Herbert Benson, *Timeless Healing* (New York: Fireside, 1996), 273.

119   *The Life and Death of a Neuron.*

120   *Social Anxiety, Chemical Imbalances in the Brain, and Brian Neural Pathways and Associations: What Does It All Mean?* Social Anxiety Institute, Inc., 2006. Available from http://www.socialanxietyinstitute.org. (accessed July, 2006).

121   See http://www.taubtherapy.com. (accessed May, 2006).

122   Shenk, 122-130.

123   Ibid., 125.

124   Ibid., 19–20.

125   Michael Castleman, et al, *There's Still a Person in There* (New York: The Berkeley Publishing Company, 1999), 126-144.

126   See http://www.nia.nih.gov/Alzheimers/Publications/adfact.htm and http://www.alzheimersdisease.com/info/answers/alzheimers-and-brain.jsp. (accessed May, 2006).

127   Shenk, 104.

128   Nancy Wong, *Failure to Seek Medical Advice for Early Symptoms of Alzheimer's Disease Regrettably Delays Diagnosis and Treatment,* Harris Interactive. Available from http://www.harrisinteractive.com. (accessed July, 2006).

129   Strauss, 58-59.

130   See http://www.alz.org/aboutad/stages.asp (accessed March, 2006).

131   Joanne Koenig Coste, *Learning to Speak Alzheimer's* (New York: Houghton Mifflin Company, 2003), 62.

132   Margaret Diamond, et. al., *Nurse Administers Therapy for Agitation in Elders* (Seattle, WA: de Tornyay Center for Healthy Aging, University of Washington School of Nursing, 2006).

133   Coste, 72-76.

134   Strauss, 114-115.

135   Castleman, 169

136   Phyllis Porter, M.A., "Early Brain Development" *Educarer* (January 10, 2006). Available from http://www.educarer.com/brain. (accessed July, 2006).

137   Strauss, 55-58.

138   Castleman, 170.

139   See www.alz.org/aboutad/stages.asp. (accessed June, 2006).

140   See http://www.feldenkrais.com or http://www.feldenkrais-method.org. (accessed June, 2006).

141   See http://www.inawareness.com. (accessed June, 2006).

142   Karma is defined as "(the result of) action or inaction" and encompasses the "cycle of cause and effect." Also known as "the universal law of consequence." In human terms, all choices and actions in one's life "create past, present and future experiences." "Karma is simply the golden rule: what you give out is what you receive." Available from http://en.wikipedia.org/wiki/Karma. (accessed August, 2006).

143   A stupa is a monument, often white and bell-shaped monument, sometimes the size of a three story building, which is a shrine in the Buddhist tradition. During a prayer ritual, saffron is thrown at the monument staining it yellow. See http://en.wikipedia.org/wiki/Stupa. (accessed September, 2006).

144   See http://www.geocities.com/Athens/Ithaca/9012/Salute_to_the_sun.htm. (accessed August, 2006).

145   Lansing Barrett Gresham and Julie J. Nichols, Ph.D., *Ask Anything and Your Body Will Answer* (Salt Lake City: NoneTooSoon Publishing, 2000), 14.

146   Valerie Hunt, *Infinite Mind* (Malibu, California: Malibu Publishing Co., 1989), 87. "Many of the experiences that we casually attribute to mind are clearly brain functions: reflexes and responses to material reality that are recorded in and recovered from the brain. Other experiences and capacities such as thought, insight, imagination, and soul seem to be properties of the higher mind."

147   See http://en.wikipedia.org/wiki/kirlian_photography. (accessed August, 2006).

148   Ayya Khema, *Being Nobody, Going Nowhere* (Boston: Wisdom Publications, 1987), 9.

149   Khema, 11.

150   Gresham, 76.

151   Ibid., 10.

152   *Therapeutic Touch Defined.* Available from http://www.therapeutictouch.org/what_is_tt.html. (accessed June, 2006).

153   Paul Dong and Aristide H. Esser, Chi Gong (New York: Marlowe & Company, 1990), 63.

154 David Eisenberg, M.D., *Encounters with Qi* (New York: W.W Norton & Company, Inc., 1995), 43.

155 Dong, 24.

156 Ibid., xxv. "Long spelled *ch'i or chi* (Wade-Giles romanization system) but in the modern pinyin romanization system rendered *qi*." Two different spellings for the same concept. I am choosing 'chi' because I think I can pronounce it.

157 Eisenberg, 44.

158 Dong, 62-63.

159 Andrew Weil, M.D., *Spontaneous Healing* (New York: Fawcett Columbine, 1995), 207.

160 Dong, 66-69.

161 Eisenberg, 43-45.

162 Dong, 66.

163 Eisenberg, 48.

164 Ibid., 50.

165 Dong, xxii.

166 Ibid., 39.

167 Ibid., 13.

168 Dong., 125.

169 Ibid., 40.

170 Ibid., 161.

171 Dong., 35.

172 Choa Kok Sui, *Pranic Healing*, xxiv.

173 Ibid., xvi.

174 Ibid., 16.

175 Choa Kok Sui, *Pranic Healing*., 18.

176 Ibid., 4.

177 Ibid., 5 and 52-55. There are seven major chakras. The First Chakra, Basic or Root, at the base of the spine; Second Chakra, Sex, lower abdomen; Third Chakra, Solar Plexus, stomach; Fourth Chakra, Heart, in front of and behind the heart; Fifth Chakra, Throat, center of throat; Sixth Chakra, Third Eye, forehead; Seventh Chakra, Crown, top of head. Each chakra is linked to a part of the physical body and also to a spiritual and an emotional component. There are also many smaller minor chakras and even smaller mini chakras. See also Caroline Myss, PhD., *Anatomy of the Spirit* (New York: Three Rivers Press, 1996), 68-70.

178 Choa Kok Sui, *Pranic Psychotherapy* (York Beach, Maine: Samuel Weiser, Inc., 1993), 25.

179 Choa Kok Sui, *Pranic Healing, xxx.*

180 Levine, Peter, PhD., *Waking the Tiger, Healing Trauma* (Berkeley, California: North Atlantic Books, 1997), 8.

181 Benson, 16-17.

182 Levine, 16.

183 Ibid., 16-19.

184 Ibid., 20-21.

185 David Servan-Schreiber, M.D., Ph.D., *Healing Without Freud or Prozac: Natural Approaches to Curing Stress, Anxiety and Depression Without Drugs and Without Psychoanalysis* (London: Rodale, Ltd., 2003), 90-91.

186 Hunt, 108.

187 Maggie Phillips, *Finding the Energy to Heal* (New York: W.W. Norton & Company, Inc., 2000), 22, 47, 52.

188 Ibid., 190.

189 Levine, 39.

190 Phillips, 50.

191 Ibid., 183.

192 Fritjof Capra, *The Tao of Physics* (New York: Bantam Books, 1980), 117.

193 Bill Moyers, *Healing and the Mind* (New York: Doubleday, 1993), 177-193.

194 Lynne McTaggart, *The Field* (New York: HarperCollins Publishers, 2002), 31.

195 See http://library.thinkquest.org/3487/qp.html. (accessed July, 2006).

196 See http://www.journey-to-success.com/Wave_Particle_Duality_qp.html. (accessed July, 2006).

197 See http://library.thinkquest.org/3487/qp.html. (accessed July, 2006).

198 McTaggart, 11.

199 Ibid., 44.

200 Ibid., 26.

201 See http://www.journey-to-success.com/Wave_Particle_Dualtiy_qp.html. (accessed July, 2006).

202 See http://library.thinkquest.org/3487/qp.html. (accessed July, 2006).

203 See http://www.calphysics.org/zpe.html. (accessed July, 2006).

204 Philip Yam, *Scientific American* (December 1997): 82-85.

205 See http://www.calphysics.org/zpq.html. (accessed July, 2006).

206 Hunt, 33.

207 McTaggart, 200.

208 Capra, 117-118.

209 Choa Kok Sui, *Pranic Healing, 5.*

210 Sue Ann Bowling, "Talking to Plants," *Alaska Science Forum,* (September 7, 1987), 837.

211 Larry Dossey, *Healing Words* (New York: Harper Paperbacks, 1997), 267.

212 Hunt, 149.

213 McTaggart, 138.

214 Ibid., 194.

215 Hunt, 266.

216 Dong, 54.

217 Judith Orloff, M.D., *Intuitive Healing* (New York: Times Books, 2000), 174-175.

218 Hunt, 267.

219 Thomas Hanna, *Somatics* (Reading, Massachusetts: Perseus Books, 1988), 19-21.

220 Kylea Taylor, *The Ethics of Caring* (Santa Cruz, California: Hanford Mead, 1995), 12.

221 Dossey, *Healing Beyond the Body,* 189-190.

222 Attention Deficit Hyperactivity Disorder, a syndrome which usually manifests in children during early school ages and can continue into adulthood. See http://www.nimh.nih.gov/publicat/ adhd.cfm. (accessed June, 2006).

223 Julie Motz, *Hands of Life* (New York: Bantam Books, 2000), 186. Julie Motz reports similar experiences with patients.

224 Caroline Myss, *Anatomy of the Spirit* (New York: Three Rivers Press, 1996), 37.

225 There are four categories of brain wave states. Beta is the fastest and occurs when we are awake and active. Alpha is slower and occurs when we are resting or in repose. Theta is even slower, a trance-like state, but still conscious. The person who was daydreaming and could not remember the drive home was in theta. Slowest is delta when we are sleeping. Dreams occur in high delta. See http://www.web-us.com/ brainwavesfunction.htm. (accessed May, 2006).

226   Eric Peper, Katherine H. Gibney and Catherine F. Holt, *Make Health Happen* (Dubuque, Iowa: Kendall Publishing Company, 2002), 194.

227   Eisenberg, 197-203.

228   Lewis Mehl-Madrona, M.D., *Coyote Medicine* (New York: Fireside, 1997), 232.

229   Ibid., 276-277.

230   Candice B. Pert, *Molecules of Emotion* (New York: Scribner, 1997), 290.

231   Orloff, 173.

232   Dossey, *Healing Beyond the Body,* 190-197. Dossey also points out that many health related dreams turn out to be false alarms, a fact which could be accounted for when the self-preservation instinct is on high alert and picks up things which only might be harmful.

233   Benson, 134.

234   Ibid., 127.

235   Pert, 286.

236   Benson, 135.

237   Moyers, 157-159.

238   Ibid., 187.

239   Dossey, *Healing Beyond the Body,* 211.

240   Weil, 93-94.

241   See http://www.tm.org. (accessed August, 2006).

242   Benson, 195,199.

243   See http://www.tm.org. (accessed August, 2006).

244   Ibid.

245   Ibid.

246   See http://www.aapb.org. (accessed August, 2006).

247   Pert, 137.

248   Siegfried Othmer, "Generality and Specificity in Biofeedback," *California Biofeedback* 22(2) (Summer, 2006). Refers to Heart Rate Variability (HRV) technique which "target[s] a larger swing of respiratory sinus arrhythmia with the cycle of slow in- and out-breath. . . By doing this breath-paced forcing at the resonant frequency of the interacting blood pressure/heart rate regulatory systems one increases the oscillation of both. Called . . . parametric oscillation . . . this challenges them both into more harmonious interaction. Better self-regulation of both ANS and heart function ensues."

249   Ibid.

250   Pert, 186-187.

251 Ibid., 293-296. It is most helpful if the exhale is double the time of the inhaled breath.

252 Thich Nhat Hanh, *Mindfulness of Breathing* (Plum Village, France, July 24, 1998).

253 Interview with Alexandra DeAvalon, Avalon, A Place for Body and Spirit, School of Massage, 1280 Boulevard Way, Suite 214, Walnut Creek, California 94595(June 23, 2006). See http://www.avalon.name. (accessed October, 2006). "For example we have a calming posture called 'child pose' (on the floor kneeling down, head to the floor, arms behind feet). This posture slows down the heart, the breath and the pressure on the abdomen, completely slowing everything down. It gives the feeling of being held and nurtured. Certain fluids are released into the brain to calm the mind."

254 Ibid., Alexandra DeAvalon.

255 "Biofeedback: The Yoga of the West," Elda Hartley, producer, Hartley Film Foundation, Cat Rock Road, Cos Cob, Connecticut, 06807 (1997).

256 Pert, 293.

257 Khema, 14.

258 Ibid., 13.

259 His Holiness the Dali Lama and Howard C. Cutler, M.D., *The Art of Happiness* (New York: Riverhead Books, 1998), 44-46.

260 Moyers, 126.

261 Pert, 285-289.

262 Benson, 134-135.

263 C.S. Lewis, *Miracles: A Preliminary Study* (New York: The MacMillan Company, 1962), 168.

264 Dossey, *Healing Words*, 141.

265 Lewis, 168.

266 Terry Matz, Director of the Church, St. Teresa of Avila. Available from Catholic Online. www.catholic.org/saints/saint.php?saint_id=208. (accessed July, 2006).

267 *The Holy Bible,* Matthew 8:5-13.

268 Hans A Baer, *Biomedicine and Alternative Healing Systems in America* (Madison, Wisconsin: University of Wisconsin Press, 2001), 121-143.

269 Benson, 227-229.

270 D. Schwender, A. Kaiser, S. Klasing, K. Peter and K. Poppel, "Midlatency auditory evoked potentials and explicit and

implicit memory in patients undergoing cardiac surgery," *Anesthesiology* 80(3) (March, 1994): 493-50. Available from http://www.ncbi.nlm.nih.gov/entrez/query.fcgi?cmd=Re trieve&db=PubMed&list_uids+8141445&dopt=Abstract. (accessed July,2006).

271   Benedict Carey, "Mental Activity Seen in a Brain Gravely Injured," *The New York Times*, CLV (53) (September 8, 2006), 696:1.

272   Myss, 33.

273   National Holistic Institute now has a similar course, and I am certain other massage schools do as well.

274   Available from Hospice and Palliative Care of Contra Costa, 3470 Buskirk Avenue, Pleasant Hill, CA 94523, (925) 887-5678.

275   Hospice and Palliative Care of Contra Costa.

276   Jo Cundrith, Hospice and Palliative Care of Contra Costa, Medicare Hospice Benefits, Department of Health and Human Services. Available from http://www.medicare.gov/ publications/pubs/pdf/02154.pdf. (accessed August, 2006).

277   Pauline, Jones, R.N., Director of Admissions, Hospice and Palliative Care of Contra Costa.

278   "Signs and Symptoms of Approaching Death," Hospice & Palliative Care of Contra Costa, 9.

279   Orloff, 51.

280   Ibid., 51.

281   Dossey, *Healing Words*, 293-323.

282   Ibid., 245-248.

283   Motz

284   Orloff, 168-172.

285   Peper, 198.

286   Moyers, 329-330.

287   Mehl-Madrona, 283.

288   Ibid., 261.

289   Ibid., 250.

290   Mehl-Madrona., 249.

291   Mario Varvoglis, Ph.D., *Psychic (Distant) Healing,* Parapsychological Association. Available from http://www. parapsych.org/pshychic_healing.htm. (accessed August, 2006).

292   Baer, 122-126. Spiritualism "teaches that disembodied spirit continues to live on after death and that mediums are able to communicate with spirits who can assist mortals in addressing everyday concerns." Nineteenth century Spiritualism "supported social reforms" and tended to try to build a congregation, but in the twentieth century it has turned to focus more on the individual.

293   Baer, 122-126.

294   Shenk, 93.

295   S.G. Urba, "Nonpharmacologic pain management in terminal care," *Clinics in Geriatric Medicine* 12(2) (May, 1996): 301-11.

296   Weil, 53.

297   Phillips, xi.

298   Dossey, *Healing Words*, 49.

299   Hand and foot reflexology works on the principle that points on the hand and foot correspond to points on the body, and working on or holding those points translates to that part of the body.

300   P. Sansone and L. Schmitt, "Providing tender touch massage to elderly nursing home residents: a demonstration project," *Geriatric Nursing 21*(6) (Nov-Dec, 2000): 303-8.

301   M. Rowe and D. Alfred, "The effectiveness of slow-stroke massage in diffusing agitated behaviors in individuals with Alzheimer's disease," *Journal of Gerontological Nursing* 25(6) (June, 1999): 22-34.

302   Motz, 80.

303   Sansone, 303-8.

304   Motz, 80.

305   Moyers, 157.

306   Dossey, *Healing Words*, 289-291.

307   Orloff, 191.

308   *Public Policy & Aging Report.*

309   Taylor, xix.

Selected Bibliography

AARP. *Normal Reactions to Loss*. Available from http://aarp.org/
families/grief_loss/a2004-11-15-reactions.html.

Abraham, Ivo, Melissa M. Bottrell, Terry Fulmer and Mathy D
Mezey. *Geriatric Nursing Protocols for Best Practice*. New
York: Springer Publishing. 1999.

Alvord, Lori Arviso, M.D. and Elizabeth Cohen Van Pelt. *The
Scalpel and the Silver Bear*. New York: Bantam Books, 2000.

American Association of Homes and Services for the Aging.
Available from http://www.2.aahsa.org.

American Geriatrics Society. *Geriatrics Review Syllabus* 5th ed. New
York: American Geriatrics Society, 2004.

Arizona Community Foundation. *Communities for All Ages Gather
Youth and Seniors from across Arizona*. Arizona Community
Foundation (March 24, 2004). Available from http://www.acf.
org.

Baer, Hans A. *Biomedicine and Alternative Healing Systems in
America*. Madison, Wisconsin: University of Wisconsin Press,
2001.

Ballentine, Rudoph, M.D. *Radical Healing*. New York: Harmony
Books, 1999.

Benson, Herbert. *Timeless Healing*. New York: Fireside, 1996.

Butler, Robert N., M.D., Lawrence K. Grossman, and Mia R.
Oberlink, eds. *Life in an Older America*. New York: The
Century Foundation Press, 1999.

Caldwell, Barbara. "Certificate of Need Regulation in the Nursing Home Industry: Has It Outlived Its Usefulness?" *American Society of Health Economists* (June, 2006). Available from http://healtheconomics.us/conference/2006/abstracts/topics-in-health-care-organizations/certificate_of_need_regulation_in_the_nursing_home_industry_has_it_outlived/.

Capra, Fritjof. *The Tao of Physics*. New York: Bantam Books, 1980.

Carper, Jean. *Your Miracle Brain*. New York: HarperCollins, 2000.

Carstensen, Laura, et al. *Practical Handbook of Clinical Gerontology*. Thousand Oaks, CA: Sage Publications, Inc., 1996.

Castleman, Michael, et al. *There's Still a Person in There*. New York: The Berkeley Publishing Company, 1999.

Charness, Neil. *Age, Technology, and Culture: Gerontopia or Dystopia.*, Washington, D.C.: National Academy on an Aging Society and The Gerontological Society of America, 2005.

Choa Kok Sui. *Pranic Healing*. York Beach, Maine: Samuel Weiser, Inc., 1990.

Choa Kok Sui. *Pranic Psychotherapy*. York Beach, Maine: Samuel Weiser, Inc., 1993.

Coste, Joanne Koenig. *Learning to Speak Alzheimer's*. New York: Houghton Mifflin Company, 2003.

Dali Lama, His Holiness and Howard C. Cutler, MD. *The Art of Happiness*. New York: Riverhead Books, 1998.

Diamond, Margaret, et. al. Nurse Administers Therapy for Agitation in Elders. Seattle, WA: de Tornay Center for Healthy Aging, University of Washington School of Nursing, 2006.

Dong, Paul and Aristide H. Esser. *Chi Gong*. New York: Marlowe & Company. 1990.

Dossey, Larry, M.D. *Healing Beyond the Body*. Boston: Shambhala Publications, Inc., 2001.

Dossey, Larry, M.D. *Healing Words*. New York: Harper Paperbacks, 1997.

Eisenberg, David M., M.D. *Encounters with Qi*. New York: W.W. Norton & Company, Inc., 1995.

Fadiman, Anne. *The Spirit Catches You and You Fall Down*. New York: Farrar, Straus and Giroux, 1997.

Federal Interagency Forum of Aging-Related Statistics. *Older Americans 2004: Key Indicators of Well-Being*. Available from http://www.agingstats.gov/chartbook2004/healthstatus.html.

Feldenkrais, Moshe. *The Potent Self*. San Francisco: Harper, 1992.

Gimbel, Theo. *Healing with Color and Light*. New York: Fireside, 1994.

Greenhalgh, Susan. *Under the Medical Gaze*. Berkeley:University of California Press, 2001.

Gresham, Lansing Barrett and Julie J. Nichols, Ph.D. *Ask Anything and Your Body Will Answer*. Salt Lake City: NoneTooSoon Publishing, 2000.

Grossman, Lawrence K. *The Media's Role: Life in an Older America*. New York: The Century Foundation Press, 1999.

Hammer, Russell D. Ph.D. *"What Can My Baby See?"* Parents' Press (November, 1990).

Hanna, Thomas. *Somatics: Reawakening the Mind's Control of Movement, Flexibility, and Health*. Reading, Massachusetts: Perseus Books, 1988.

Harrington, Charlene, Ph.D., James H. Swan, Ph.D., John A. Nyman, Ph. D. and Helen Carrillo, MS. "The Effect of Certificate of Need and Moratoria Policy on Change in Nursing Home Beds in the United States." *Medical Care* 35:6 (June, 1997).

Huber, Julia. *The New Old – How Baby Boomers are Redefining Retirement*. AARP Policy and Research (July, 2004). Available from: http://www.aarp.org/research/reference/boomers/a2004-07-22-globalperspectives.html.

Hunt, Valerie. *Infinite Mind*. Malibu, California: Malibu Publishing Co., 1989.

Khema, Ayya. *Being Nobody, Going Nowhere*. Boston: Wisdom Publications, 1987.

Levine, Peter, PhD. *Waking the Tiger, Healing Trauma*. Berkeley, California: North Atlantic Books, 1997.

Lewis, C.S. *Miracles: A Preliminary Study*. New York: The MacMillan Company, 1962.

Luhrmann, T.M. *Of Two Minds*. New York: Vintage Books, 2000.

Mazey, M. et al. *Geriatric Nursing Protocols for Best Practice*, 2nd ed. New York: Springer Publishing Company, 2003.

McTaggart, Lynne. *The Field*. New York: HarperCollins Publishers, 2002.

Mehl-Madrona, Lewis, M.D. *Coyote Medicine*. New York: Fireside, 1997.

Merck Institute of Aging and Health. *Nurse's Notes for Healthy Aging*. Available from http://wwwmiahonline.org/resources/ nursenotes/articles/01_10_05.grief_reactions.html.

Merck Institute of Aging and Health. *The Sate of Aging in America*. Washington, D.C.: The Gerontological Society of America, 2003. Available from http://www.agingsociety.org/agingsociety/ pdf/state_of_aging_report.pdf.

Morgan, Marlo. *Mutant Message Down Under*. New York: HarperCollins, 1991.

Motz, Julie. *Hands of Life*. New York: Bantam Books, 2000.

Moyers, Bill. *Healing and the Mind*. New York: Doubleday, 1993.

Myss, Caroline, PhD. *Anatomy of the Spirit*. New York: Three Rivers Press, 1996.

National Academy on Aging. *Facts on Long Term Care*. Washington, D.C.: National Academy on Aging, 1997.

National Academy on Aging. *What Are the Attitudes of Young Retirees and Older Workers?* Washington, D.C.: National Academy on Aging, February, 2001. Available from http://wwwagingsociety.org/agingsociety/pdf/aarp5.pdf.

National Academy on Aging. *Who are Young Retirees and Older Workers?* Washington, D.C.: National Academy on Aging, June, 2000. Available from http://www.agingsociety.org/agingsociety/pdf/aarp1.pdf.

National Academy on an Aging Society. *Public Policy & Aging Report.* Washington, D.C.: National Academy on an Aging Society and the Gerontological Society of America, 2005.

National Institute on Aging. National Institutes of Health, Public Health Services. U.S. Department of Health and Human Services, April 25, 2006. Available from http://www.nia.nih.gov/Alzheimers/Publications/adfact.htm#Contents.

National Institute of Neurological Disorders and Stroke. *The Life and Death of a Neuron.* Bethesda, MD.: NIH Publications, 2005.

Noekler, Linda S. *Training Direct Care Workers for Person-Centered Care, Public Policy and Aging Report.* Washington D.C.:

National Academy on an Aging Society and the Gerontologiacal Society of America, 2005.

Orloff, Judith, M.D. *Intuitive Healing.* New York: Times Books, 2000.

Othmer, Siegfried. "Generality and Specificity in Biofeedback." *California Biofeedback* 22(2) (Summer, 2006).

Peper, Eric, Katherine H. Gibney and Catherine F. Holt. *Make Health Happen.* Dubuque, Iowa: Kendall Publishing Company, 2002.

Pert, Candice B. *Molecules of Emotion.* New York: Scribner, 1997.

Phillips, Maggie. *Finding the Energy to Heal.* New York: W.W. Norton & Company, Inc., 2000.

Porter, Phyllis, M.A. "Early Brain Development." *Educarer* (January 10, 2006). Available from http://www.educarer.com/brain.

Radin, Lisa and Gary Radin, eds. *What If It's Not Alzheimer's?* New York: Prometheus Books, 2003.

Rix, Sara E. "The Older Worker in a Graying America." *Life in an Older America*. New York: The Century Foundation Press, 1999.

Rossman, Martin L., M.D. *Guided Imagery for Self-Healing*. Tiburon: H.J. Kramer, Inc. and New World Library, 2000.

Rowe, M. and D. Alfred. "The effectiveness of slow-stroke massage in diffusing agitated behaviors in individuals with Alzheimer's disease." *Journal of Gerontological Nursing* 25(6) (June, 1999).

Ruffin, Novella J. Ph.D. *Understanding Growth and Development Patterns of Infants*. Blacksburg, VA: Virginia Polytechnic Institute and State University, 2001.

Sansone, P. and L. Schmitt. "Providing tender touch massage to elderly nursing home residents: a demonstration project." *Geriatric Nursing* 21(6) (Nov-Dec, 2000).

Sapolsky, Robert M. *Why Zebras Don't Get Ulcers*. New York: W. H. Freeman and Company, 1998.

Schwender, D., A. Kaiser, S. Klasing, K. Peter and K. Poppel. "Midlatency auditory evoked potentials and explicit and implicit memory in patients undergoing cardiac surgery." *Anesthesiology* 80(3) (March, 1994). Available from http://www.ncbi.nlm.nih.gov/entrez/query.fcgi?cmd=Retrieve&db=PubMed&list_uids+8141445&dopt=Abstract. *The Secret Life of the Brain*. Available from http://www.pbs.org/brain.

Servan-Schrieber, David, M.D., Ph.D. *Healing Without Freud or Prozac: Natural Approaches to Curing Stress, Anxiety and Depression Without Drugs and Without Psychoanalysis*. London: Rodale, Ltd., 2003.

Shenk, David. *The Forgetting*. New York: Anchor Books, 2003.

Slater, Philip. *Pursuit of Loneliness*. Boston: Beacon Press, 1976.

Smith, Linda Tuhiwai. *Decolonizing Methodologies*. New York: Zed Books, Ltd., 1999.

Social Anxiety Institute. *Social Anxiety, Chemical Imbalances in the Brain, and Brain Neural Pathways and Associations: What Does It All Mean?*

Social Anxiety Institute, Inc. 2006. Available from http://www.social anxietyinstitute.org.

Stafford, Philip B. *Creating Lifespan Communities, Public Policy and Aging Report*. Washington D.C.: National Academy on an Aging Society and The Gerontological Society of America, 2005.

Stone, Robyn I. *Long-Term Care of the Elderly with Disabilities*. New York: Milbank Memorial Fund, 2000.

Strauss, Claudia J. *Talking to Alzheimer's*. Oakland, CA.: New Harbinger Publications, Inc., 2001.

University of Toronto. Quality of Life Research Unit, Center for Function and Well-Being. Available from http://www.utoronto. ca/qol/seniors.htm.

Upledger, John, D.O., O.M.M. *A Brain Is Born*. Berkeley: North Atlantic Books, 1996.

Upledger, John, D.O., O.M.M. *Your Inner Physician and You*. Berkeley: North Atlantic Books, 1997.

Urba, S.G. "Nonpharmacologic pain management in terminal care." *Clinics in Geriatric Medicine* 12(2) (May, 1996).

Varvoglis, Mario Ph.D. *Psychic (Distant) Healing*. Parapsychological Association. Available from http://www.parapsych. orgpshychic_healing.htm.

Viorst, Judith. *Necessary Losses*. New York: The Free Press, 1986.

Watson, Wendy L. *Aging is a Family Affair*. Brigham Young University, Family Studies Center. Available form http://family center.byu.edu/Columbus.aspx?id=47.

Weil, Andrew, M.D. *Spontaneous Healing*. New York: Fawcett Columbine, 1995.

Weinstein, Michelle. *Laughter is the 'Best Medicine' for Your Heart*. Baltimore, MD: The University of Maryland Medical Center. Available from http://www.umm.edu/features/laughter.htm.

Wong, Nancy. *Failure to Seek Medical Advice for Early Symptoms of Alzheimer's Disease Regrettably Delays Diagnosis and Treatment*. Harris Interactive. Available from http://www. harrisinteractive.com.

Yam, Philip. *Scientific American* (December, 1997).

Resources

Aging

Administration on Aging
U.S. Health & Human Services
200 Independence Avenue, SW
Washington, DC 20201
800-677-1116
http://www.aoa.gov
Government agency that provides nationwide resources for the elderly. Topics include health, care, finance and legal issues among others. Links to other agencies.

Alliance for Aging Research
2021 K Street, NW
Suite 305
Washington, DC 20006
202-293-2856
http://www.agingresearch.org
Non-profit advocacy organization that intends to "promote medical and behavioral research into the aging process." Access to press articles on the latest research.

American Association of Retired Persons (AARP)
601 E Street, NW
Washington, DC 20049
888-687-2277
http://www.aarp.org
"A non-profit membership organization of persons 50 and older dedicated to addressing their needs and interests." Member benefits include health insurance, travel discounts, financial services and legal services.

American Society on Aging
833 Market Street
Suite 511
San Francisco, CA 94103
800-537-9728
http://www.asaging.org
A non-profit organization made up of multidisciplinary professionals who are "bound by a common goal: to support the commitment and enhance the knowledge and skills of those who seek to improve the quality of life of older adults and their families." Offers educational programs, training, conferences and publications on the subject of aging.

National Council on Aging
300 D Street, SW
Suite 801
Washington, DC 20024
202-479-1200
http://www.ncoa.org
A non-profit organization that offers educational programs aimed at helping seniors with issues such as Medicare, benefits, healthy aging, employment and civic engagement. Acts as advocate for seniors and maintains a network of collaborating organizations.

National Institute on Aging
Building 31, Room 5C27
31 Center Drive, MSC 2292
Bethesda, MD 20892
800-222-2225
http://www.nia.nih.gov
Government agency formed to "provide leadership in aging research, training, health information dissemination, and other programs relevant to aging and older people." Research funding.

Alzheimer's and other specific diseases

Alzheimer's Association
225 N. Michigan Ave., Fl. 17
Chicago, IL 60601
800-272-3900
http://www.alz.org
A non-profit volunteer organization with local chapters nationwide.
It offers information and support for families and caregivers of
Alzheimer's sufferers. Services include 24/7 Helpline, CareFinder™,
Safe Return®, extensive library dedicated to Alzheimer's disease and
a journal. Also funds research.

Alzheimer's Disease Education and Referral Center
P.O. Box 820
Silver Spring, MD 20907
800-438-4380
http://www.alzheirmers.nia.nih.gov
Government agency created to "compile, archive, and disseminate
information concerning Alzheimer's disease for health professionals,
people with AD and their families, and the public." Information
center that answers questions, publications, referrals to local support
groups.

Alzheimer's Foundation of America
322 8th Ave., 6th Fl.
New York, NY 10001
866-232-8484
http://www.alzfdn.org
A non-profit organization whose mission is "to provide optimal
care and services to individuals confronting dementia, and to their
caregivers and families – through member organizations dedicated
to improving quality of life." Services include a hotline, educational
materials and workshops, counseling, resources and referral centers,
support groups for different stages of dementia, respite programs and
early detection screenings.

Alzheimer's Resource Room
Alzheimer's Demonstration Project
Administration on Aging
Washington, DC 20201
202-357-3452
http://www.aoa.gov/alz/index.asp
Government agency providing resources to elders, caregivers, professionals and providers who are dealing with Alzheimer's disease.

American Parkinson Disease Association
135 Parkinson Avenue
Staten Island, NY 10305
800-223-2732
http://apdaparkinson.org
A non-profit organization dedicated to "ease the burden and find a cure" for Parkinson's disease. It has nationwide local chapters that focus on education, information, support and fund raising.

Creutzfeldt-Jakob Disease Foundation
P.O. Box 5312
Akron, OH 44334
800-659-1991
http://www.cjdfoundation.org
A non-profit organization founded to "support families and loved ones touched by CJD." Provides medical information, on-line chat room and resources.

Lewy Body Dementia Association
P.O. Box 11390
Tempe, AZ 85284
480-894-1100
http://www.lewybodydementia.org
A non-profit organization "dedicated to raising awareness of Lewy Body disease, assisting caregivers and families and encouraging scientific advancements." Caregivers' Hotline.

Pick's Disease Support Group
info@pdsg.org.uk
http://www.pdsg.org.uk
A support group offering information and contacts regarding this
frontal lobe dementia.

Medical and Health Care

American Geriatrics Society
The Empire State Building
350 Fifth Avenue, Suite 801
New York, NY 10118
212-308-1414
http://www.americangeriatrics.org
A non-profit organization which is an "association of geriatrics health
care professional, research scientists, and other concerned individuals
dedicated to improving the health, independence and quality of life
of all older people." Provides education on health care concerns of
older people, including Medicare information and a physician referral
service.

Eldercare Locator
800-677-1116
http://www.eldercare.gov/Eldercare/Public/Home.asp
Government agency connecting "those who need assistance with
state and local area agencies on aging and community-based
organizations that serve older adults and their caregivers". A variety
of languages are offered.

Institute of Noetic Sciences
101 San Antonio Road
Petaluma, CA 94952
707-775-3500
http://www.ions.org
A non-profit membership organization "that conducts and
sponsors leading-edge research into the potentials and powers of
consciousness – including perceptions, beliefs, attention, intention,
and intuition." Educational programs and publications; co-sponsors
events around the world.

Meals on Wheels Association of America
203 S. Union Street
Alexandria, VA 22314
703-548-5558
http://www.mowaa.org
A non-profit organization that focuses on serving nutritious meals
to seniors in need. They also give cash grants to local senior meal
programs throughout the country.

National Policy and Resource Center on Nutrition and Aging
Florida International University, OE 200
Miami, FL 33199
305-348-1517
http://nutritionandagign.fiu.edu
Government sponsored center acts as a clearinghouse for information,
meetings, events and publications on nutrition, physical activity
and aging. Comprehensive list of research, reports and resources.
"Creative Solutions" section showcases successful local programs.

Natural Standard
1 Broadway, 14th Floor
Cambridge, MA 02142
617-758-4270
http://www.naturalstandard.com
An impartial service which "aggregates and synthesizes data on
complementary and alternative therapies." Analysis provides
"objective, reliable information that aids clinicians, patients, and
healthcare institutions to make more informed and safer therapeutic
decisions."

Touch Therapies

Alexander Technique

Movement based therapy that releases inhibition and tension and makes room for learning. In the process, self-awareness is increased. The Complete Guide to the Alexander Technique
http://www.alexandertechnique.com
Information; find a teacher or a course.

American Massage Therapy Association

500 Davis Street, Suite 900
Evanston, IL 60201
877-905-2700
http://amtamassage.org
A non-profit organization that "represents more than 55,000 massage therapists in 27 countries. AMTA works to establish massage therapy as integral to the maintenance of good health and complementary to other therapeutic processes." Find a massage therapist search or find a massage school.

Cortical Field Re-Education

A somatic movement therapy that promotes health and well being.
http://www.thecfrsite.com
History and list of practitioners.

CranioSacral Therapy

A light-touch therapy that improves the central nervous system.
Available through:
Upledger Institute
11211 Prosperity Farms Road, Suite D-325
Palm Beach Gardens, FL 33410
800-233-5880
http://www.upledger.com
A "health resource center dedicated to the advancement of complementary and innovative techniques." Classes for healthcare practitioners. Find a therapist search option.

Feldenkrais Method

An awareness therapy promoting health and healing. "My inmost belief is that, just as anatomy has helped us to get an intimate knowledge of the working of the body, and neuroanatomy an understanding of some activities of the psyche, so will understanding of the somatic aspects of consciousness enable us to know ourselves more intimately." Moshe Feldenkrais

International Feldenkrais Federation

http://feldenkrais-method.org
"The coordinating organization of most Feldenkrais Guilds and Associations and other key Feldenkrais professional organizations worldwide." Provides list of associations in many countries.

Feldenkrais Guild of North America

3611 SW Hood Ave. Suite 100
Portland, OR 97239
503-221-6612
http://www.feldenkraisguild.com

Integrated Awareness

A "process of self-healing through self-discovery." Workshops and individual sessions.
http://www.inawareness.com
List of classes, events and practitioners.

Reiki

A hands-on "Japanese technique for stress reduction and relaxation that also promotes healing."
The International Association of Reiki Professionals
603-881-8838
http://www.iarp.org
Reiki news, find a class or practitioner.

Rosen Method

Gentle touch that releases muscle tensions and aids the person in "becoming more aware of his/her body and internal experience."
The Rosen Institute
800-893-2622
http://www.rosenmethod.org
Descriptions, training centers, find a practitioner.

Somatic Experiencing/Trauma Healing
Provides tools for healing trauma. Information, resources and a list
of practitioners.
Foundation for Human Enrichment
7102 La Vista Place, Suite 200
Niwot, CO 80503
303-652-4035
http://www.traumahealing.com

There are many excellent massage therapy schools in
the US. Here are two with which the author has had
personal experience:

National Holistic Institute
5900 Hollis St., Ste. Q
Emeryville, CA 94608
510-547-6442
http://www.nhimassage.com
Comprehensive career massage therapy program with hands-on
practical experience. Four locations, all in California.

McKinnon Institute
2940 Webster Street
Oakland, CA 94609
510-465-3488
http://www,mckinnonmassage.com
Flexible massage therapy program that encourages "safe, competent,
caring touch" in a positive environment. Continuing education.

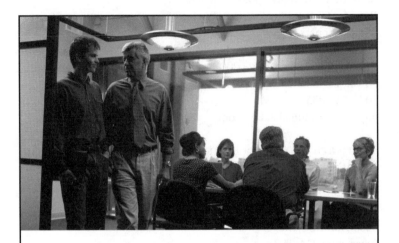

SHARE THIS MESSAGE

Bulk Discounts
Discounts start at a low number of copies, ranging from 30% to 50% off based on the quantity chosen.

Custom Publishing
Would you like a private label? or a customization to suit your needs. We could even highlight specific chapters.

Sponsorship
Would you like to sponsor this book? It's a great way to advertise your product or service in a unique way!

Dynamic Speakers
Authors are available to you, to share their expertise at your event!

Call LifeSuccess Publishing at 1-800-473-7134 or email
info@lifesuccesspublishing.com for more information

OTHER BOOKS FROM LifeSuccess Publishing

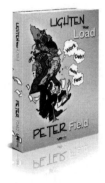

Lighten Your Load

Peter Field

ISBN # 1-59930-000-1

Your Doctor Said WHAT?
Exposing The Communication Gap

Terrie Wurzbacher

ISBN # 1-59930-029-X

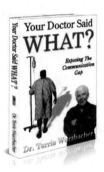

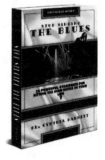

Stop Singing The Blues
10 Powerful Strategies For Hitting The
High Notes In Your Life

Dr Cynthia Barnett

ISBN # 1-59930-022-2

OTHER BOOKS FROM LifeSuccess PUBLISHING

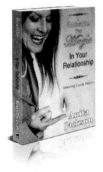

Rekindle The Magic In Your Relationship
Making Love Work

Anita Jackson

ISBN # 1-59930-041-9

Wellness Our Birthright
How to give a baby the best start in life.

Vivien Clere Green

ISBN # 1-59930-020-6

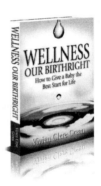

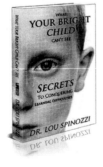

What Your Bright Child Can't See
Secrets To Conquering Learning
Difficulties

Dr Lou Spinozzi

ISBN # 1-59930-033-8

NOTES

NOTES

NOTES

NOTES

NOTES

NOTES

NOTES

NOTES